The Patient's Guide to Urology
(Plumbing Problems in Layman's Terms)

G. Mark Seal, M.D., F.A.C.S.

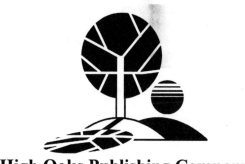

High Oaks Publishing Company
Toledo, Ohio

First Edition
First Printing

Library of Congress Cataloging-in-Publication Data
Seal, G. Mark
The patient's guide to urology (plumbing problems in layman's terms)/ by
        G. Mark Seal, M.D., F.A.C.S.
        p. 272.
        Includes index, glossary, and illustrations.
        ISBN 0-9645773-0-5 (Cloth)
        ISBN 0-9645773-1-3 (Paper)
        95-94094

FOREWORD

In an economic and social construct, patients are consumers of medical goods and services. In this time of "consumer advocacy", Dr. Mark Seal has written an outstanding piece in the name of "patient advocacy".

In the past years, a doctor-patient relationship found the former to be the active party, and the latter the passive one. One does not have to be too old to remember the crusty, old curmudgeon Dr. Kildare (played by Lionel Barrymore) in his wheelchair uttering pronouncements such as: "Do this. I know best. Trust me." There was neither time nor inclination for dialogue or real patient instruction.

Fortunately today, there is a much more interactive process between doctor and patient. But this is highly variable. A book of this nature addresses this point. The base knowledge offered to the patient in the area of Urology is now standardized, thanks to Dr. Seal, at a very high level.

The reader is offered current, detailed information on the pathophysiology of each Urologic disease and a rational basis for the choice of therapy. It is ideally suited for patients, family practitioners, nurses, and paramedical personnel alike. Indeed, Urologists would do well to have this in their offices, so they may refer patients for instruction in a particular problem area.

Dr. Seal has made good use of consultants so that the material herein is scientifically current and correct; but it is written in a clear, understandable style. All things considered, this is a timely and useful piece for all those who must deal with Urologic problems, be they patients or those ministering to them.

John P. Donohue, M.D., F.A.C.S.
Distinguished Professor and Chairman
Department of Urology
Indiana University School of Medicine
Indianapolis, Indiana

December, 1994

ACKNOWLEDGEMENTS

I would like to thank my wife, Eleanore, and my lovely children, Ryan and Allie, for their support of my writing while actively practicing medicine and trying to be a good husband and dad simultaneously.

For their technical support, I would also like to thank Mr. Dan Wiland and Mr. Ghaleb Abu Alhana. For the development of the "lap-top" computer which has made projects like mine possible, I would like to thank the brilliant people of the computer industry. The ability to take computer technology with you wherever you go, even to McDonald's® for their great coffee, is an incredible boost to efficient and creative use of time.

And finally, I would like to thank the following professors of urology, each of whom reviewed the chapters within their specific areas of expertise. I have appreciated their constructive comments and additional expertise which their comments have contributed.

John P. Donohue, M.D., F.A.C.S.
Distinguished Professor and Chairman
Department of Urology
Indiana University School of Medicine
Indianapolis, Indiana
Chapters 8, 14, and 21.

Kenneth Kropp, M.D., F.A.C.S.
Professor of Surgery and
Pediatrics
Medical College of Ohio
Toledo, Ohio
Chapters 3, 4, 13, 15, 16,and 18

Shlomo Raz, M.D.
Professor of Surgery and
Urology
University of California, Los
Angeles, School of Medicine
Los Angeles, California.
Chapters 9, 10, 11, and 12.

Martin Resnick, M.D., F.A.C.S.
Lester Persky Professor of
Urology and Chairman
Case Western Reserve
University, School of Medicine
Cleveland, Ohio
Chapters 6, 7, and 17

Stacy J. Childs, M.D.
Editor in Chief, INFECTIONS
IN UROLOGY
Medical Director, Southeastern
Research Foundation
Birmingham, Alabama
Chapters 11, 12, 20, 24, 25, 26, and 27.

Anthony Thomas, M.D.
Chief of Section, Infertility
Department of Urology
Cleveland Clinic Foundation
Cleveland, Ohio
Chapters 2, 5, 19, 22, and 23.

DEDICATION AND PURPOSE

In my specialty training of urology, I learned that if you could not verbalize the explanation of a condition or disease, you probably did not completely understand it. Becoming a teacher, whether of patients, medical students, or your peers earned esteem equal to that of other aspects of your progress in becoming a surgeon. This book reflects that valuable priority and is dedicated to the patients, nurses, medical students, residents, and faculty who served and continue to serve as my educators in my surgical training and practice.

Physician training is, in large part, self-directed and self-perpetuated. Particularly during internship and residency, the residents and students, overseen by faculty members, prepare and present a majority of the individual case studies and teaching conferences. The ability to explain becomes crucial. Unfortunately, many physicians forget that those countless hours of preparation must be used later in communicating to their patients.

For those patients whose problems are discussed within the following pages, I hope that this book will help them understand their conditions, not only for the peace of mind better understanding can bring, but also to allow the formulation of useful and important questions to ask to their physicians. These pages seek neither to manage the readers' problems, nor is it possible to be 100% "up to date" as changes in technologies and treatments occur on almost a daily basis. The intent in this book is not self-treatment, and any interpretation as such may quite frankly yield a disastrous outcome for the patient.

Properly read, this book offers a better understanding of the principles in the functioning of the normal genital and urinary tracts, the common malfunctions resulting from disease, and the principles of treatment. If we stay to the course as writer and reader, these pages will be useful for the readers long after they were first read.

TABLE OF CONTENTS

TOPICS ON THE PENIS

TOPICS ON THE PROSTATE GLAND

TOPICS ON THE URINARY BLADDER

TOPICS ON THE KIDNEY

TOPICS ON THE MALE GENITALIA

TOPICS ON INFECTION

TOPICS ON MEDICINE TODAY

GLOSSARY AND INDEX

TABLE OF ILLUSTRATIONS

TOPICS ON THE MALE GENITALIA

TOPICS ON INFECTION

All illustrations by Mr. Mark Valenti and Ms. Lori Hepler.

The illustrations were produced through the utilization of freehand sketching and computer illustration and enhancement. All freehand illustrations were scanned at 300dpi at 75% of their original size utilizing a UMAX 630c scanner with propietary software. Each illustration was bitmapped edited for style consistency and enhancement and stored in TIFF format for import. The illustration and enhancement software used was Micrografx Designer 3.1 and Picture Publisher 4.0 (Micrografx Inc.).

CHAPTER 1

WHAT IS A UROLOGIST?

A brief discussion of urology as a surgical speciality.

A urologist is first a physician, second a surgeon, and third, a surgeon specializing in disorders of the genitourinary tract. Specifically, a urologist's area of expertise falls within diseases of the adrenal glands, kidneys, ureters, bladder, and the male organs (scrotum, penis, testicles, prostate, seminal vesicles). Obviously, this system does not function in isolation; all of our systems, i.e. the nervous system, digestive system, and circulatory system, interact in very intimate fashion.

Many disciplines overlap with the urologic specialty, and therefore, several problems may be treated by either a urologist or another surgeon or physician, i.e. a gynecologist can also treat urinary incontinence of females, a general surgeon may also treat hydrocoeles or hernias in males, or an endocrinologist may also evaluate and treat a patient for the medical management of kidney stones.

Therefore, any urologic evaluation begins with a patient's complete history and physical examination to alert the urologist to any problems or conditions outside of the urinary tract which may be part of the specific complaint. It is important that a urologist draw upon an understanding of all the systems in coming to a diagnosis and treatment of what appears to be a specific urologic disease.

CHAPTER 2

IMPOTENCE

The causes and treatments of erection problems of the penis.

There's the old story about the man who came to the hospital in a tuxedo on the day of his surgery. When asked "Why?", he responded, "My doctor told me I am 'impotant' so I want to dress 'impotant'."

DEFINITION

"Impotence" simply means the inability to sustain an erection satisfactory for intercourse. It is to be distinguished from erogenous stimulation (sensation), from orgasm (climax), and from ejaculation (jettison of sperm and associated secretions)--for, while each of these occur during "normal" sexual activity, each is a different physiologic (bodily) process and each may be impaired separately, as well as in combination. "Normal" sexual activity occurs with each of these different functions contributing cooperatively

Our discussion will center upon only impotence for now. The other processes which cause sexual impairment will be discussed later in this chapter.

Impotence actually refers to the result of a spectrum of problems which urologists and therapists prefer to term "erectile dysfunction." While it is estimated that 10 million American men are truly impotent, another 10 million suffer in varying degrees with erectile dysfunction. Very infrequent is the situation like turning off a light switch--that is, sudden and complete loss of the ability to have erections. Rather, the usual course of erectile dysfunction is a progression over several months to years with, perhaps, times when it is noticeable interspersed between times of obviously successful sexual activity. The two most common initial symptoms are the inability to sustain an erection to completion of the act and/or a loss in the rigidity of the erection with difficulty upon intromission (penetration).

Let's now discuss the anatomy and how normal erections occur.

ANATOMY

The penis consists of several circular layers of tissues surrounding three tubular chambers (See Figure 2-1). Examined in cross-section, as you would

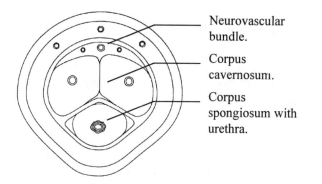

Neurovascular bundle.

Corpus cavernosum.

Corpus spongiosum with urethra.

Figure 2-1: The penis in cross-section.

the loaf of fresh bread from your local bakery, it is more triangular than perfectly round. On the underside of the penis is the tubular chamber (the corpus spongiosum) which houses the urethra, the tube which conducts the urine and ejaculate out. On the top are the two other chambers (corpora cavernosa), side by side, which house the erectile tissue, the sponge-like tissue which becomes engorged when an erection occurs. In the groove between the two corpora cavernosa is the neurovascular bundle (nerve and blood vessel package) which provides sensation and blood supply to the penis.

The erectile tissue is like a sponge--made up of millions of microscopic blood vessels. Tiny valves are present which control the flow of blood through these vessels. Each valve and the blood vessel itself is controlled by a network of tiny microscopic nerves and local chemical releases directed by these nerves to allow tumescence (erection) and detumescence (deflation or resolution of an erection) to occur at the proper time and for the appropriate duration. It's not hard then to understand that any disease process which affects blood vessels, i.e. atherosclerosis, or nerves, i.e. diabetes mellitus will profoundly alter this function. These nerves originate in the sacral (lowest) area of the spine and are part of the autonomic (automatic) nervous system called the parasympathetic nervous system which also controls the bladder.

Erections occur as a result more of a slowing of the blood flow out of the penis than any dramatic increase of flow into the penis. There is an increase of blood flow which begins the process but reaches a steady state. Think of your garden hose attached at the house. You turn the hose on which increases the flow initially, but soon reaches a flow with water running at a constant rate. When you step on the hose, partially occluding it, it becomes more stiff or rigid between the house and where your foot is placed. The valves in the erectile tissue slow the flow of blood out of the penis, causing the spongy tissue to fill with blood within the confines of the corporal chambers, inflating them to a point of rigidity, much like the water fills the hose until it can hold no more and the pressure within the hose rises. For the erection to go down, appropriate messages are sent through the nerves and local chemical mediators to release the valves. There's a purge of blood from the penis back into the generel circulation, and detumescence (deflation) is completed.

The corpora cavernosa, or two erectile chambers of the penis, separate once they are in the trunk of the body (See Figure 2-2). This allows the urethra to come up between them and join to the prostate gland, but it also allows them to abut or push against the ischium bone on each side. The next time you're undressed (both men and women), feel up high where your leg joins your trunk on the inner aspect of your thigh. You'll feel the ischium.

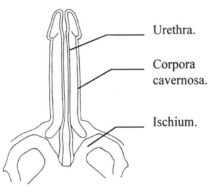

Urethra.

Corpora cavernosa.

Ischium.

Figure 2-2: The penis in its long axis.

The importance of the abutment is that this prevents the penis "retreating" during intercourse. In other words, with the penis erect, this abutment serves

7

to allow deep penetration for ejaculation important in procreation, and of course, may enhance a satisfying experience for both sexual partners.

With this overview of the erection process, let's look at those aspects of body functioning which directly affect normal potency.

Vascular:
The first critical function is that provided by healthy blood vessels (vascular). As described previously, millions of tiny blood vessels housed in the chambers of the penis become engorged with blood, like a dry sponge swelling with water, resulting in an erection. Therefore, any disease which affects blood vessels, like arteriosclerosis, "hardening of the arteries", will affect this ability. Smoking and its affects on the vascular system is the most commonly linked exogenous (substance brought into the body by eating, inhaling, or absorbing through the skin) factor. The risk of developing a blockage of 50% or more in the larger penile artery is 15% higher for men who have smoked a pack a day for five years than for non-smokers. The percentage doubles to more than 30% for one pack-a-day smokers with a 10 year habit, and it quadruples for those with 20 years of pack-a-day smoking. Hypertension (high blood pressure) is commonly associated with impotence because of its toll on the vessels over many years time. Occasionally in the context of treating high blood pressure, some gentlemans will complain that the partial erectile ability they once had has been completely lost. Certain groups of medications are associated with this side-effect, particularly those which directly dilate the blood vessels. Most physicians are well acquainted with this patient complaint and have at their disposal groups of medications, i.e. calcium channel blockers, which are as good in controlling the blood pressure with a minimum effect upon potency.

Occasionally, the larger blood vessels delivering blood to the penis from within the pelvis of the male are affected, and the sponge network itself is intact. Liken this to a tree with healthy limbs and branches but a problem develops with the trunk or roots. The best example is trauma, i.e. a pelvic fracture (broken bones of the pelvis) where the blood vessels are severed as they pass through the floor of the pelvis into the penis. Leriche Syndrome, extensive hardening of the arteries of the pelvic arteries including those which feed the penile arteries, is yet another example of problems with the trunk or main delivery system.

One final vascular or blood flow problem deserves our attention. As opposed to the affects of high blood pressure affecting the delivery (or inflow) of blood to the penis for erections to occur, this occurs on the outflow side of things and is called Venous Leak Syndrome. With venous leak, as the turgor (pressure) in the penis goes up, there is a spontaneous release or purge, and the penis immediately goes down. This is a particularly frustrating condition because the gentleman is able to begin sexual activity, often including insertion and beginning intercourse, but then the penis spontaneously softens. The treatment is difficult, surgically identifying the leak and surgically tying it off, or often having to resort to a penile implant.

Another condition of erectile dysfunction associated with penile curvature is called Peyronie's Disease (See Chapter 5).

Nerves:
The second critical function is an intact nervous system. Any diseases which take their toll on nerves will diminish the ability to control the millions of flow in the blood vessels of the penis.. The tiny nerves involved in this function are part of the autonomic (or automatic) nervous system--controlling a whole host of the body's function which occur automatically, without a thought, i.e. the ability to urinate by the bladder. The nerves originate in the sacral or lowest part of the spinal cord and are called the Parasympathetic Nervous System. There are nerves going to and from the spinal cord controlling this function. The brain in a very complex manner coordinates, processes, and commands this ability--but let's simplify things. True to many women's ideas of men, the penis wants to be erect constantly. The brain and upper spinal cord above the reflex arc (consisting of a nerve out to its point of activity and a nerve back to the central nervous system, See Figure 9-5) in the lowest portion of the spinal cord are constantly suppressing this activity. Similar to the contraction of the bladder with urination, the brain " allows" (and in the context of erogenous activity "encourages") an erection to occur. If this suppression is lost but the lower mechanism or reflex arc remains intact, reflex erections can occur. We see these for instance with high level spinal cord injury patients wherein stimulation, even non-sexual like the movement of a leg or the stimulation of the nerves of the skin by bathing, results in an uncontrolled erection which generally is not satisfactory for sexual activity as it is not timely and not usually sustained.

Large nerves, in a relative sense when compared to those within the penis itself, may be injured as they exit the floor of the pelvis next to the prostate gland--either in trauma or in the context of surgery, i.e. for cancer of the prostate gland or for some large bowel (colon) and rectal procedures. This type of injury begins with the surgery or trauma. However, the impotence need not be permanent. Oftentimes, after a period of 3 to 6 months, the erectile activity does return. As our understanding of the nerve and blood supply to the penis has become more sophisticated, so have our surgical procedures which previously almost uniformly destroyed structures critical to the maintenance of potency. However, in performing cancer surgery, there clearly should be no compromising of the goal of the surgery--to remove the cancer--in order to preserve potency. To quote an old adage,"You can't take it with you!".

Psychological:
Thirdly, in order to function normally in a sexual way, there clearly has to be reasonable psychological stability. If there are serious disturbances either within the man or in the relationship, it would not be surprising that sexual dysfunction, perhaps even impotence, could occur. The classic situation is the forty year-old gentleman who fears factory layoffs, is somewhat bored in his marriage of nearly 20 years, and has just found out his teenager is using drugs. Life has just closed in on him from all directions. Generally, unless truly severe, the gentleman will demonstrate normal ability or potential ability by the evaluation. In other words, we will most often exclude"organic impotence" by testing, to be described later in the chapter. This gentleman's problem is just as real to him as to the gentleman who cannot perform because of a prostate operation; it's just for a different reason. He cannot perform in times of intimacy because of his psychologic pressures which have been internalized to a destructive degree. Additionally, anxiety created by anticipating that he is going to have difficulty even prior to engaging in sexual activity, promulgates a downward spiraling of emotions called "performance anxiety". Much like the athlete going into a contest fearing injury, the distraction in and of itself contributes to causing that which is most feared. Obviously, counseling is the treatment of choice for this gentleman, hopefully involving a caring and supportive spouse or sexual partner.

Hormonal:
The fourth major functional consideration is that of hormonal balance. Historically, this was the only arena of treatment available to the urologist-- prescribing testosterone, the male hormone. However, as our understanding of the mechanisms of erection have expanded, so have the treatments. True hormonal dysfunction encompasses the smallest percentage of patients with impotence. Generally, these patients can perform, as proven by occasional successful intercourse. However, they seldom engage in sexual activity because of lack of libido (sex drive). Frequently, it will be the spouse or

sexual partner who voices the complaint and is concerned about the lack of interest in sexual activity. Physical exam frequently is normal, but can on occasion display small or absent testicles. A blood test, the serum testosterone level, will be low, and measurement of other hormonal blood tests, LH and FSH, may point to a pituitary problem (a small gland in the brain) which directs testicle function. (See Male Infertility, Chapter 23). This group of problems will be treated by testosterone supplementation if the primary cause of the hormonal problem cannot be otherwise addressed.

EVALUATION

The evaluation starts with a complete history and physical examination, including psychosocial aspects of the patient's behavior and relationships. As noted above, even a seemingly unrelated illness, i.e. a thyroid disorder, may come to bear upon the problem. After this review, screening bloodwork to assure good hematologic and physiologic balance will be checked. Additional more specific testing for hormonal balance, i.e. serum testosterone, LH, FSH, and prolactin may be checked.

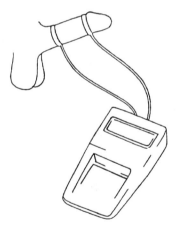

Figure 2-3: The nocturnal penile tumescence monitor.

The most definitive test is called N.P.T., nocturnal penile tumescence--based on fact that every man who has normal erectile ability has several erections at night during sleep, associated with deep sleep. It's too bad because they're wasted. Remember, erections occur as a release phenomena; that is, as the brain relinquishes full control during deep sleep, the penis seizes the opportunity to become erect. To measure this ability, the patient places two rubber band-like devices around the penis: one at the junction near the scrotum and one near the corona, the groove at the head of the penis (See Figure 2-3). These are strain gauges and record in a little microcomputer (about the size of an electric razor) to which they are attached and which is left on the patient's nightstand at home. As the erection occurs, the bands are stretched, and this is recorded. Previous measurements of the penile girth without erection allow us to place in a percentage form what the predicted values of a "great" erection would be, and it is against this value that the patient's results are scaled (See Figure 2-4).

The information in this test tells us not only whether or not erections occur, but also provides us with some assessment of the quality of those erections, enabling us to tailor treatments to the patient's degree of impairment. Also, even if the tracings are normal, this can be a source of reassurance to the patient and might make him much more receptive to psychological evaluation and treatment.

AMBULATORY RIGIDITY AND TUMESCENCE MONITOR

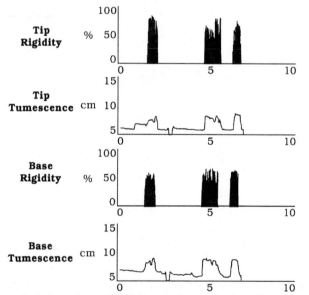

Figure 2-4: Sample tracing for normal nocturnal penile tumescence.

Penile dopplers measure blood flow through the penis and can be indexed against blood pressures in the arm to assess the severity of the blockage(s). Arteriograms and corporal studies, using contrast injection in a radiology suite in the hospital, are rarely performed to assess blood vessel problems. Neurologic evaluation and testing may be ordered if the problem is thought to fall within conditions of nerve disorders.

TREATMENT

If there are contributing factors from other aspects of the patient's medical condition(s) which could be altered, then this serves as a starting point of treatment, i.e. if certain blood pressure medications are thought to be worsening the situation. Assuming that the condition is thought to be strictly genitourinary, the first line of treatment is a group to medications which are designed to improve blood flow through small blood vessels. One such medication is Trental®, pentoxifylline. Yocon®, or yohombine, is a medication of unknown action which some physicians have used with limited success.

The next line of treatment is injection therapy. In this treatment, the patient learns to inject a small amount of medication into the corpora of the penis, flooding it with chemical mediators causing erection (See Figure 2-5).

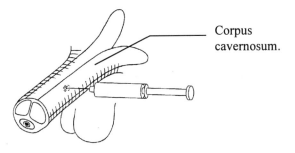

Corpus cavernosum.

Figure 2-5: Self-injection treatment for impotence.

Erections will last for 15 to 60 minutes usually. Four to six visits to the urologist's office allow a mastery of the technique and an adjustment of the medication required for the desired result. From that point the patient is provided with a prescription, usually for 12 to 15 pre-filled syringes, to be used on a once or twice per week basis and never to be injected more than once per 24 hour period. The medication may be papaverine alone, papaverine with phentolamine, or certain prostaglandins. The advantages and disadvantages of each as well as the dosage is explained and tailored to the patient, and most urologists providing these prescriptions will have the patient sign a contract of sorts which outlines the agreed upon dosages and maximum frequencies of usage.

While on the surface this may seem not a satisfactory option, consider the following scenario. A couple anticipates sexual activity after a nice evening out with friends. Prior to engaging in sexual activity, most would excuse themselves to the privacy of the restroom. During that time, the gentleman gives himself an injection. The couple then engage in foreplay. During that time of 10 or 15 minutes or so, the medication has the opportunity to provide an erection satisfactory for intercourse as the woman's secretions ready the vagina for intercourse. Intercourse is completed and the penis will detumesce (go down) as the medication is metabolized. If used in this fashion, the use of injection therapy need not be disruptive to relatively normal sexual activity and allows the use of the patient's "own machinery" for as long as possible.

An additional treatment is a suction-type (vacuum-constriction) device which assists in the engorgement of the penis. This is teamed with the use of a band or ring which is rolled off of the suction device into position at the base of the penis, to slow the outflow of blood, thus sustaining the erection (See Figure 2-6). When the erection is no longer desired, the band is removed and the erection promptly resolves. While used satisfactorily by many couples, of all treatments this is the most intrusive at the time of intimacy.

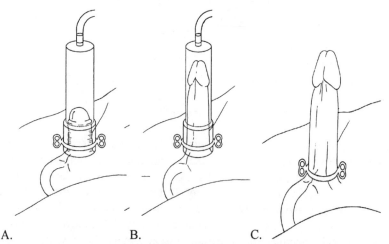

A.   B.   C.

Figure 2-6: Vacuum constriction treatment for impotence.

14

The most invasive treatment is the insertion of the penile implant. This prosthetic device, inserted into each corpus cavernosum (therefore, two are placed--one in each corpus) to provide rigidity adequate for intercourse. It must be stressed right from the outset that these devices will NOT alter sensation, neither enhancing nor diminishing it; they will NOT alter ejaculation, neither improving nor destroying that ability; and finally, they will NOT alter orgasm, neither enhancing nor diminishing it. They simply provide an erection which will allow intercourse. In doing so they will generally enhance the sexual experience of the patient, but penile prostheses do not alter directly the other components of the sexual experience except erection.

The surgical insertion generally takes about 1 to 1 ½ hours and can be performed using regional anesthesia. The incision can be like a circumcision (circular just behind the corona or head of the penis), a small incision on the underside of the penis at the penoscrotal junction (the joining of the penis with the scrotum), or at the junction of the penis at the pubic bone (the hard bone above the genitalia). The choice of incision is dependent upon which type of prosthesis is chosen and surgeon preference.

While there are several different "re-creations of the wheel" from different manufacturers, in general the prostheses comes in three different types. The first type is called a semi-rigid prosthesisand is a malleable (bendable) silastic (plastic) device which when inserted gives the penis a permanent erection (See Figure 2-7). It is bendable, and therefore is disguised by use of

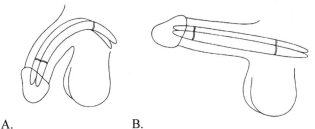

A.   B.

Figure 2-7: Semi-rigid penile prosthesis.

tighter underwear which bend the penis against the body. The advantage of this type is that it has no moving parts, i.e. pumps or inflatable chambers to break or wear, and requires no hand dexterity or learning curve to function adequately. For this reason as an example, the semi-rigid prosthesis is a good prosthesis for the stroke patient who has been left with impaired hand dexterity. The down side is obviously that the penis appears and feels erect all the time and may restrict some activities due to embarrassment, i.e. public showering.

The second type of prosthesis is the inflatable penile prosthesis (See Figure 2-8). In this device, fluid (usually normal saline--salt water) is pumped from

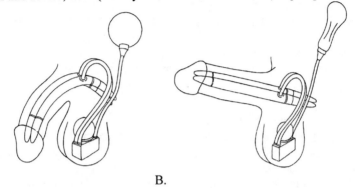

A.   B.

Figure 2-8: Inflatable penile prosthesis.

a reservoir into the cylinders which have been placed in each corpus cavernosum. The pump is placed in the scrotum and is easily disguised there. I tell gentlemans it's "like having a third testicle!" Squeezing the pump draws fluid through the connection tubing from the reservoir, which has been placed in the abdomen above the pubic bone in front of the bladder, to the cylinders. After sexual activity, a release valve is activated on the pump and the fluid is returned to the reservoir. The disadvantages of this type of prosthesis include: these are the most costly; they have the highest mechanical failure rate (approximately 5% because they are assembled in components); they require good hand dexterity, a learning curve for use, and a fairly sophisticated patient for acceptance. The advantages are the excellent functional penis they afford for sexual activity and the excellent detumescence (deflated penis) provided.

The third type of prosthesis is actually a blending of the two previously described. This is called a "self-contained" inflatable prosthesis (See Figure 2-9). The device does inflate and deflate, and it is inserted in the corpora similar to the semi-rigid. The fluid is pumped from the surrounding larger chamber down a more central pylon, yielding its rigidity. When the erection is no longer desired, a release valve within the device allows the normal

16

saline to return to the outer larger chamber reducing the pressure and rigidity of the central pylon.

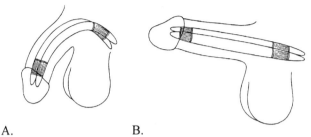

A.   B.

Figure 2-9: Self-contained, inflatable penile prosthesis.

The insertion is easier than the multi-component type, but the working of the prosthesis requires a longer learning curve and more dexterity because of the positioning of the pump. Some complain that the deflated prosthesis does not leave them with a penis which looks entirely deflated. Nonetheless, thousands of these have been inserted by urologists with great satisfaction recorded by a majority of patients.

Another surgical option, for use in a very select group of patients, are vascular (blood vessel) surgeries designed either to improve inflow or to impede outflow. These involve either "harvesting" small veins to re-vascularize (blood vessels reconstruction, either arteries or veins) the penis or re-routing the arteries to the penis. These are highly specialized procedures performed by urologists with special interests and training in impotence, and most of these procedures involve the use of microscopic techniques.

Peyronie's Disease represents a unique condition and is discussed in its own chapter (See Chapter 5).

PARTNER SATISFACTION

Studies indicate that the sexual partner's satisfaction rate is very high if the spouse or partner is allowed to participate in the process from its outset, including the psychological evaluation and patient and partner preparation which is usually in order before the insertion of the penile implant. Frequently, the spouse or partner would be advised to seek a gynecologic evaluation prior to resuming intercourse so as to anticipate any problems which would preclude a satisfying experience for the woman. For instance, there may be the need to medically treat atrophic vaginitis (a condition wherein the vagina contracts and the lining becomes quite dry) and perhaps even provide some vaginal dilation prior to resuming intercourse, particularly if it has been a substantial period of time since intercourse was last experienced.

OTHER SEXUAL DISORDERS

As mentioned in the introduction of this chapter and repeated in the goals of prosthetic surgery, impotence denotes only an erection problem. Other disorders might include a reduction or loss in sensation, i.e. the peripheral neuropathy experienced by diabetics, for which little can currently be done. There may be problems with ejaculation, which is controlled by the sympathetic nervous system. In some cases, this can be treated by the use of alpha-adrenergic preparations, i.e. frequently used over the counter cold preparations like Actifed or Sudafed, just prior to sexual activity. Orgasm is the perception of the "sexual high". Problems in this area generally fall within the psychologic treatment realm.

Greater accuracy in the diagnosis combined with increasing treatment options offer most patients reasonable expectations to successfully overcome erectile dysfunction and/or other sexual disorders.

CHAPTER 3

CIRCUMCISION

Surgical removal of the foreskin of the penis.

The surgical procedure to remove excess foreskin from the penis is called circumcision, a procedure depicted in drawings in the ancient Egyptian tombs (See Cover.) which has served in religious ceremonies as well. Today, although simple to perform, this procedure remains debated regarding its medical necessity. It has shifted in and out of favor among pediatricians, obstetricians, and urologists through the years.

In deciding whether or not any surgical procedure should be performed, one must consider its purposes. Circumcision is not a necessary procedure for the newborn. It is performed, however, with very specific and clear goals in mind.

First, all surfaces of the body must be periodically examined. Lack of visual access to a part of the body eliminates or lessens the opportunity to detect problems earlier. In a condition called phimosis, the foreskin tightens over the end of the penis such that it cannot be retracted to clean or exam the glans penis (head of the penis). The risk of malignancy of the penis is extremely low in the U.S. (0.3 to 1.1/100,000 men per year) and cannot be used alone as an indication to perform circumcision. However, the inability to examine the glans penis (head of the penis) and meatus (urethral opening) is a reason to perform circumcision.

Circumcision makes the hygiene of male genitals more easily accomplished. Many parents become lax at retracting the foreskin to cleanse and to dry when bathing. Over time, the penis does tend to develop phimosis. I've seen this frequently even with the most meticulous and caring parents. When the infant grows into a toddler he becomes very ticklish and then care becomes even more difficult. Again, this does not make circumcision necessary, but parents should be aware that there will be extra time and work involved in the care of the uncircumcised child.

The third consideration is one of recurrent infection. I have rarely seen a balanitis (infection on the head of the penis) in a circumcised child, but I have seen many in the uncircumcised. This usually relates to hygiene. This can be painful and disturbing to the child and parents. Retrospective studies have shown the incidence of urinary tract infections to be nearly 20 times greater in the uncircumcised male than in the circumcised. On a recurrent basis, infections can be disruptive to toilet-training and, in severe cases, may cause a scarring of the head of the penis leading to a blockage at the opening (meatus) called meatal stenosis. As adults, studies associating sexually transmitted diseases with the avoidance of circumcision have not been scientifically validated.

A fourth consideration is simply cosmetic. If an aesthetic choice of penile appearance leads to circumcision, the parents should not be made to feel guilty for making such a decision. It is far preferable to do this as an infant than when the boy is one or two years old. In fact, I have discouraged circumcision in older children unless there are more clear cut (no pun intended), medically compelling reasons and, if the choice is made, frequently have attempted to time the circumcision with another necessary surgical procedure, i.e. myringotomy tubes (ear tubes for recurrent middle ear infections, placed by ear, nose and throat specialists).

Any surgical procedure carries certain inherent risks, i.e. the risk associated with anesthesia, with bleeding, with infection, and with pain. Opponents of circumcision can use these as arguments against circumcision. Each risk, while significant in a very few cases, is minimal and can be outweighed if:

      1.) the reasons for proceeding are clear,
      2.) the timing of the procedure is optimal, and
      3.) the attentiveness to detail in making the experience as favorable as possible for the child is assured.

Circumcision may not be advisable for a child who is not well, i.e. who has chronic illness such as bleeding disorders, etc., and, of course, any genital deformity which would require further reconstruction, i.e. hypospadias (See Chapter 4), in which the opening for urination does not reach the tip of the penis.

We've discussed the reasons to proceed with circumcision. A particularly frustrating experience for parents is, having made and acted upon the decision to have their infant circumcised, to find a year or two later having it suggested that it be "revised" for various reasons, i.e. the development of phimosis or an "unsuitable cosmetic result". There has been a trend over the last 10 years to not perform a complete circumcision upon newborns. What we are seeing, though, are many young boys who have the appearance of not having been circumcised at all. Newborn circumcisions are done with a device called a Plastibell® or Gomco® clamp (See Figure 3-1). It basically has a shield or cup to protect the head and then crushes and severs the excess skin, fusing it at its line of excision. The device is excellent for its intended purpose and can yield an excellent result in skilled and experienced hands. Unfortunately, because they are slightly unpleasant to perform, are not that intellectually challenging for the operator, and, in training programs in obstetrics, pediatrics, and family practice are considered drudgery by the residents, the least experienced personnel perform them. The parents should question the qualifications of whomever will perform the surgery.

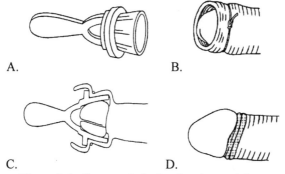

A.   B.

C.   D.

Figure 3-1: Gompco® device for circumcision.

Timing can make all the difference in the world. By age 2, a young boy has integrated the penis well into his psyche. The emotional upset for penile surgery, whether it be circumcision or other more extensive procedures such as hypospadias repairs (to place the penile meatus at the tip for better urination), increases as the child gets older. Therefore, this work is most optimally completed by age 2. Anesthetic safety approaches that of an adult after the first year. Therefore, for elective circumcision or penile surgery, many urologists recommend doing the work between the ages of 1 and 2.

Attentiveness to detail for the child includes much more than simply what's done at the operating table once the child is asleep. It includes a friendly receiving and preparation area where the child can wait with his parents-- away from the hectic and concerning pace of most preoperative preparation areas. It includes friendly and nurturing staff. It includes a readiness of the operating room, including the anesthetist, to promptly get the child comfortable and asleep when he's taken from his parents. It includes, prior to awakening from the general anesthetic, the use of local, long-acting anesthetic agents like Marcaine® or Sensorcaine®, either injected into the penis to numb it entirely for a period of 8 to 12 hours at the completion of the surgery or a caudal block by injecting into the low back. It includes nurturing recovery room staff and a quiet corner for the child to be held and hugged after he emerges from the anesthetic. And finally it includes a safe and prompt return of the child to those in whom he finds greatest security--his parents.

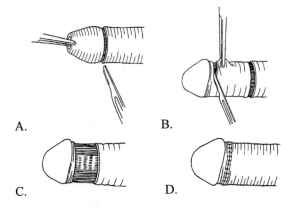

A. B.

C. D.

Figure 3-2: Surgical circumcision.

Technically, the procedure is fairly simple to perform (See Figure 3-2). The excess skin is excised and a closure is performed to assure a good cosmetic result, eliminating redundancy of skin and assuring good alignment of the median raphe, the line running up the middle of the underside of the penis. Many urologists carefully reconstruct the frenulum, the web of tissue near the head of the penis, on its underside in the middle. This area will become an important erogenous area later. Also a good closure will fashion the layers under the skin to accentuate the corona or groove around the head of the penis to assure a good cosmetic appearance. Suture which dissolves is used, therefore no stitches will need removal. Unless there are extenuating circumstances, i.e. an abnormal bladder, a catheter or tube into the bladder is not necessary. Follow-up is generally simple--only an appointment or two over the first several weeks post-operatively to assess wound healing.

Wound care is simple--as with any simple incision or laceration. Each time the diaper is changed or a few times per day in the toilet-trained boy, a simple cleanse with a warm washcloth or a cottonball with an application of a small amount of antibiotic salve should suffice.

A transient change in urinary habits is sometimes reported by parents, i.e. the child may wet the bed or have some daytime accidents. This observation has no anatomic basis, but represents a short-term psychologic upset by virtue of having undergone penile surgery. Obviously, the older child would be more likely to experience this. Long term or permanent change or upset is exceedingly rare.

Adult circumcision is performed for the same reasons as with the child: to provide access to all surface area for self-examination and hygiene, to minimize the risk of recurrent penile infections, to lessen risk for certain venereal communicable diseases, and for cosmetic reasons. The procedure is performed in similar fashion and can be performed under a penile block (numbing of the penis only), in the outpatient setting, and with the use of long-acting anesthetic agents to ensure several hours of reasonable post-operative comfort. There is no doubt that the procedure is better tolerated by children, but many of the "horror stories" told of adult circumcision simply are that--stories.

CHAPTER 4

HYPOSPADIAS

A common problem in formation of the opening at the tip of the penis.

This is a congenital (developmental) condition of the penis in which the opening of the urethra, called the meatus, fails to position itself all the way to the tip of the penis. It varies in severity, ranging from an opening on the glans penis (head of the penis), which is not out on the very tip yielding a slit or groove-like appearance, to a meatus which is positioned within the folds of the scrotum.

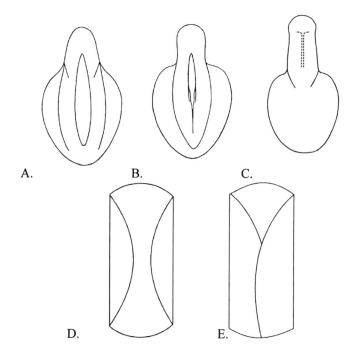

Figure 4-1: Formation of the shaft of the penis

This formation of the genitals is under the direction of testosterone or the male hormone. Conversion of testosterone to another similar chemical compound is required for the formation of the male genitals--and this conversion occurs only in those cells which are destined to become the scrotum and penis. The urethra, or conduit which carries the urine the length of penis, is formed in the womb by the first 12 weeks of development.This occurs by the folding over of the sides of the penis lengthwise and then fusing in the middle, much like rolling up the edges of a soft taco (See Figure 4-1). The end of the penis also develops a dimple which becomes deeper and deeper, much like pushing your finger into a blown up balloon (See Figure 4-2).

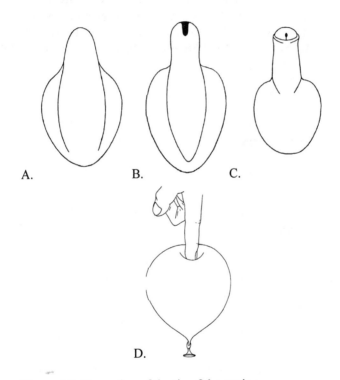

A.   B.   C.

D.

Figure 4-2: Formation of the tip of the penis.

The rolling in proceeds from the scrotum (which was also formed by fusing in the center of the two sides) outward until it meets the dimple end on yielding an intact urethra to the tip of the penis (See Figure 4-3). Failure of the urethral folds not to complete their migration outward will result in hypospadias for about 1 out of every 300 live births.

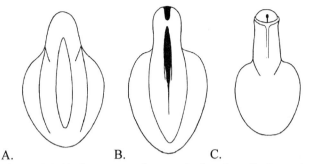

A.   B.   C.

Figure 4-3: Fusing to complete urethral and penile formation.

Two other anomalies of the penis are associated with hypospadias: dorsal hood and chordee. With a dorsal hood, the foreskin of the hypospadic penis may also fail to migrate the entire way out especially on the underside (urethral) of the penis. This gives the appearance of alot of skin redundancy on the top side of the penis adding to the unsightliness of the penis for the parents of the newborn. But is critically important to save this skin by not performing a circumcision. It is this skin which can be utilized later to construct a new urethra.

Chordee refers to the tipping down of the tip of the penis, like the nose of the SST (Supersonic Transport), the jet aircraft. This occurs because beyond the meatus, or opening in the hypospadic penis, is a string of scar tissue which tethers the head of the penis down (See Figure 4-4).

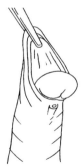

Figure 4-4: Chordee or tipping of the end of the penis and the associated dorsal hood.

This is corrected at the time of the hypospadias repair because, in addition to rendering the penis a better cosmetic appearance, it will prevent painful intercourse later by eliminating an accentuated downward curvature during erection.

Do all of these boys need surgery to correct this defect? NO. If not, then what determines which are "fixed" and which are left alone?

The goals of surgery for hypospadias are three:

1.) To allow ease in directing the urinary stream;
2.) To allow, later in life, deep intromisssion (penetration during intercourse) for deep ejaculation, thus protecting procreation; and,
3.) To improve cosmetic appearance.

1.) The ability to "direct urinary stream" simply means that the opening allows a clean exit without spray and far enough out on the penis to allow the stream to be directed by pointing the penis into a toilet. Frequently with severe chordee, the stream will spray wildly preventing any ability to control its direction. The patient is unhappy because he appears continually wet, and the family is unhappy because of the obvious mess this causes in the bathroom.

2.) The ability to father a child successfully depends upon several factors, not the least of which is the simple mechanical consideration of ejaculating in deep penetration to allow the sperm easy access to the cervix. If the meatus is closer to the scrotum, ejaculation will occur, but not into a position to allow access to the cervix and uterus. Moving the opening out helps to assure future fertility.

3.) The cosmetic consideration often becomes the most troublesome to the parents. Obviously there is considerable emotional upset for the parents submitting their 1 year old infant to surgery--of the penis, no less. If the present anatomy meets the first two goals, then the decision becomes purely one based upon cosmetic considerations.

A very unsightly dorsal hood may be treated by no more than an extensive circumcision to remove the excess foreskin on the top of the penis rendering it a normal appearance without addressing a very mild hypospadias. With significant chordee, a sizable distance between the present opening and the tip of the penis may need to be made up, accomplished through the use of the skin of the dorsal hood. Thus two cosmetic improvements are made at the same time: eliminating the curve and eliminating the mound of tissue on the top of the penis.

Three examples of the myriad of hypospadias repairs are shown below. They are demonstrations of the various techniques available based upon the severity of the deformity (from mild to severe) and surgeon preference.

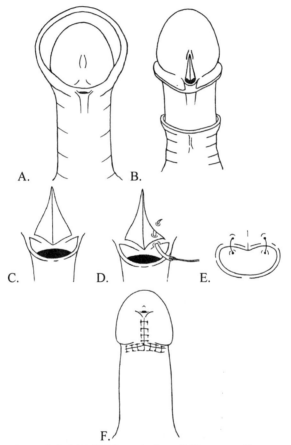

Figure 4-5: MAGPI Repair for mild hypospadias.

1.) MAGPI repair:Short for Meatal Advancement and Glanduloplasty, in essence this technique takes a slit and closes it sideways yielding the "illusion" that the opening has been advanced--used for very mild hypospadias (See Figure 4-5).

2.) FLIP-FLAP repair: Advances the tube by using a flap of skin at the meatus to construct additional length--used for lengths of less than 1.5 cm. distance (See Figure 4-6).

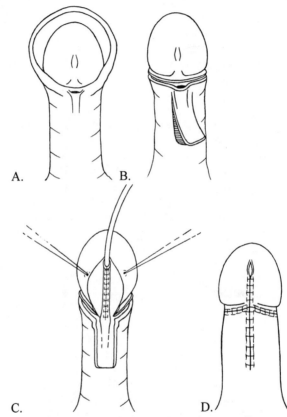

A.   B.

C.   D.

Figure 4-6: FLIP-FLAP Repair for moderate hypospadias.

3.) DUCKETT PREPUTIAL ISLAND PEDICLE FLAP: Advances the opening significant lengths (up to the entire length of the penis) by use of the redundant skin of the dorsal hood--used for more severe cases, i.e. mid-penile or even scrotal openings (See Figure 4-7).

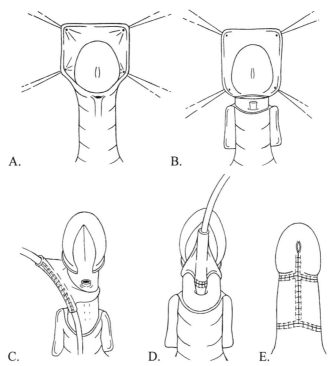

A.   B.

C.   D.   E.

Figure 4-7: DUCKETT Repair for severe hypospadias.

Hypospadias repair is best accomplished around 12 to 15 months. This allows ample growth to:

    1.) minimize the anesthetic risks (which level out at around age 12 months);

    2.) optimize the size of the penis with which to work; and,

    3.) minimize the psychologic upset to the child both in regards to integration of the penis as an important part of the male psyche and in regards to the trauma of separation from the parents.

It also is helpful to have a very "workable" penis for more effective toilet training later.

Urologists expect many questions with hypospadias referrals, and parental consternation with the decisions to be made is not uncommon. Hopefully, parents will be less upset with the deformity through a better understanding of its cause, its treatments, and have a better understanding of the goals of repair after reading this chapter.

that used for reconstruction of blood vessels by the vascular surgeons (See Figure 5-2).

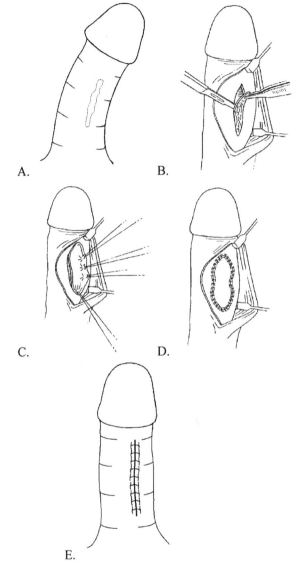

A.

B.

C.

D.

E.

Figure 5-2: Surgical excision and graft replacement technique.

The second approach is to not disturb the plaque(s) but rather to excise a wedge of tissue from the corpus cavernosum on the opposite side of the curvature, close the gap, and thereby render a straighter appearance (See Figure 5-3). The advantages and disadvantages to each of these can be discussed by the urologist, but what is absolutely key to success is that neither procedure be performed if the process is still active as indicated by pain or progressive curvature.

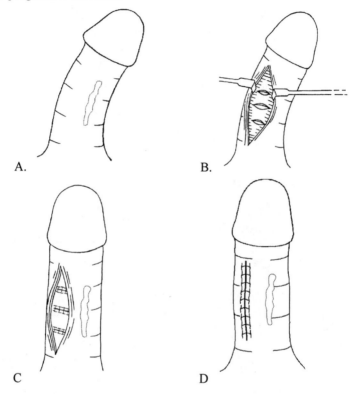

A.

B.

C

D

Figure 5-3: The Nesbitt Procedure for Peyronie's Disease.

Most urologists would wait a minimum of 6 months since the last symptom or sign of activity before proceeding with surgical correction. To assure the best surgical result, clinical photographs of the erect penis (generally taken by the patient at home) are important, and during the procedure itself, the urologist will provide the patient with a "pseudo-erection" in which normal saline is injected into the corporal bodies of the penis (See Impotence, Chapter 2) with a tourniquet positioned where the penis joins with the trunk of the body. After surgery, a period of healing is required as the tissues mature and gain elasticity. Most patients will continue to function sexually in normal fashion within approximately 6 weeks.

The previous theory that all patients who incur Peyronie's Disease will progress to impotence is not supported by the experts, nor should impotence be expected as the norm after corrective surgery. The decision to insert a penile prosthesis at the time of corrective surgery should be made based upon the patient's innate erectile ability (or inability) as documented for any patient with erectile dysfunction. What makes sense is the use of the patient's own machinery for as long as one possibly can before resorting to a prosthetic device.

CHAPTER 6

THE PROSTATE GLAND: GENERAL CONSIDERATIONS

An introduction to the prostate gland.

The prostate gland remains an enigma to many men even after some have had surgery for problems relating to it. Supposedly sinister in its purpose (because it has not been explained to the patient) and difficult to understand because of its location, the prostate gland remains a source of frustration to those who are experiencing difficulties related to it. In this chapter we will explain what the prostate gland is and where it is located. With this better understanding we will then embark upon a discussion of benign (non-cancerous) enlargement. Following that discussion we will discuss cancer of the prostate, a sometimes confusing disease even for physicians. In a later chapter, infections of the prostate will be covered.

The prostate has basically 3 functions: first, to provide a significant volume of the ejaculate; second to afford the bladder additional protection from infection; and third, much like the spine "supports" the chiropractor, the prostate gland helps to pay for urologists' kids' college educations.

As a gland, the prostate's main purpose is the production of the secretions which are critically important to fertility as they provide:

      1.) nutrients to the sperm,
      2.) an optimal chemical environment for sperm function (to be good swimmers and penetrators), and
      3.) 25 to 50% by volume of the ejaculate.

Another 50% or more is provided by the additional glands called the seminal vesicles (more on these in a minute). This bolus, or additional volume, provided by the secretions of the prostate and seminal vesicles is required for successful ejaculation or jettisoning of the sperm, which comprise only 2 to 5% by volume of the normal ejaculate.

The prostate gland also plays a role in defending the bladder from infections. It, however, may be susceptible to infections which, on occasion, can be quite severe, even life-threatening, or very prolonged and difficult to clear.

The everyday breakfast doughnut serves as a capable model for the prostate gland. The gland is roughly spherical and surrounds the urethra (the tube through which the urine passes to escape the bladder) much like a doughnut surrounds its hole (See Figure 6-1). Beginning about the size of a walnut in the young adult male, the prostate enlarges with age. The final size varies, but with some it may proceed to the size of an orange or greater. However, not only does the doughnut get bigger, but the hole in the doughnut gets smaller, often yielding the classic complaints of urine flow blockage discussed in more detail in a following chapter (See Chapter 7, Prostate Enlargement).

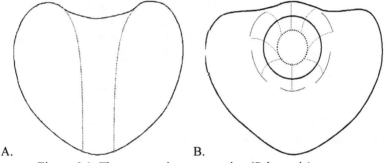

A.   B.

Figure 6-1: The prostate in cross section (Schematic).

Within the prostate are two main zones (See Figure 6-1). Since we've already used a breakfast food, let's use the analogy of the orange which you had at lunchtime. The central portion of the prostate, analogous to the fruit of the orange, is the location of the glands which manufacture the secretions and is the area which increases in size circumferentially, thus reducing the diameter of the urethra which it surrounds. The peripheral portion of the prostate, analogous to the peel of the orange, consists of compressed prostate tissue and is the location for a majority of prostate malignancies or cancers, also to be discussed in more detail to follow.

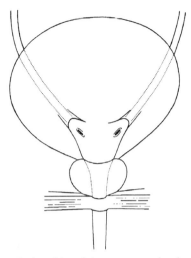

Figure 6-2: The relationship of the prostate gland and bladder.

In Chapter 9, Bladder Basics and Incontinence, the bladder is described as teardrop-shaped. In men, the prostrate surrounds the neck of the teardrop (See Figure 6-2). The prostate sits under the area of the bladder called the trigone, a triangularly shaped area at the neck of the bladder with the hole (or orifice) through which the urine coming from each kidney occupies 2 points on the triangle and the entry in the prostate being the third point on the triangle. This area has the highest concentration of nerve endings and as such may yield tremendous bladder irritation during bouts of prostate infection. The urine flows from the bladder through the prostate, then through the pelvic floor sheet of muscle, then through the urethra of the penis to exit. The prostate sits on the floor of the pelvis like your orange on the lunch table.

Well known to most army recruits and, hopefully, to most adult men over age forty, the prostate resides approximately one finger length inside the anal verge and can be felt protruding from the front wall of the rectum upon digital examination. The ability to be examined in conjunction with the peripheral location (that closest to the rectum) in a majority of cancers of the prostate, make rectal examination an imperative part of routine male physical examination.

The prostate gland is also joined by a pair of glands called the seminal vesicles. As the name "seminal" suggests (not Seminole, F.S.U. fans), these glands produce approximately 50% or more by volume of the ejaculate for similar purposes as the prostate. They are located on the top side of the prostate and are arranged much like a rabbit's ears, with the rabbit's head being the prostate (See Figure 6-3). The "ears" are directed up and actually behind the neck of the bladder. The seminal vesicles too reside on the front wall of the rectum and can occasionally be felt on rectal exam. Because of the close proximity to the prostate, occasionally the seminal vesicles may be mistaken for a lump on the prostate itself.

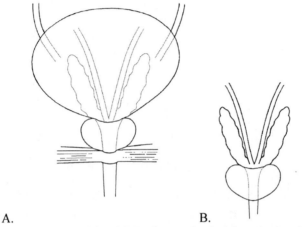

A.   B.

Figure 6-3: The relationship of the prostate gland and seminal vesicles.

Lastly, before going into a discussion of conditions of the prostate, we need to discuss the relationship of the drainage of the testicles to the prostate gland. Discussed more completely in Chapters 19 and 23 on Scrotal Concerns and Male Infertility respectively, the vas deferens (or just "vas") is the muscular tube which brings the products of the testicles (sperm and a few other products) into the channel to allow ejaculation through the urethra (See Figure 6-3). This connection, within the prostate, is called the ejaculatory duct. The vas makes a gentle arc as it sweeps through the pelvis and joins the prostate near its attachment at the floor of the pelvis in the midline (middle). The structure where this junction occurs can be seen by the urologist during cystoscopy examinations and serves as a critical landmark during endoscopic prostate surgery. The vas deferens as a connection to the scrotum also makes understandable the scrotal complaints often voiced by patients with prostate irritation or the changes in ejaculation experienced following prostate surgery.

Let's now proceed to a discussion of specific maladies of the prostate.

CHAPTER 7

PROSTATE ENLARGEMENT

Benign (non-cancerous) enlargement of the prostate.

Benign prostatic hypertrophy (BPH), or enlargement of the prostate (which is not cancer), is most common cause of urinary tract obstruction. While any abnormality of the prostate is a potential source of urinary tract blockage, BPH is the most common. The prostate increases in size from puberty until the age of 30, remaining stable until approximately age 45. At this age it undergoes benign enlargement until death.

BPH is rare before age 40, and autopsies in men over 40 show that approximately 80% have evidence of BPH, 95% by their 70's. Mean age for the detection of BPH is 65 years in Caucasians, 60 years in Negroes, and considerably lower in Orientals.

As discussed previously, while prostate gland development is relatively complex with 5 different lobes melting into one gland, it can be thought of functionally as being divided into 2 main zones. The central zone, surrounding the urethra and consisting mainly of glands which provide a majority of the ejaculate, affords some protection to the bladder from infection, As these glands enlarge, they constrict the aperture of the urethra, much like a tightening collar, resulting in symptoms of urinary blockage (See Figure 6-1, Chapter 6). The peripheral zone of the prostate is much like an orange peel, consisting of compressed fibrous and muscular prostate tissue. This peripheral zone is the location of most prostate malignancies. The plane between these two main zones provides a very important landmark for urologists during prostate surgery and will be discussed further in the context of each of the prostate surgeries.

There is considerable evidence to show that endocrine control plays the major role in BPH. This now serves as a treatment regimen for BPH and will be discussed later in this chapter. What remains unclear is the differences in incidence between races and even that between different families. I have seen many cases of sons reporting their fathers had problems with BPH as relatively young men also.

SYMPTOMS

Enlargement of the prostate, per se, causes no manifestations. It is the obstruction or blockage of the urethra (the tube connecting the bladder the outside) which causes patients to complain. As a result of the blockage, the bladder must generate higher pressures in order to urinate. The time it takes to achieve this extra pressure may be perceived as a delay in time before urination begins, or hesitancy. What stream is generated may be appreciably slower than previously, or it might be every bit as strong but requires more effort to empty. This can be best understood by thinking of the common garden hose attached to your house. With the water running, there is some pressure in the hose but what enters the hose, exits at the same rate. Now step on the hose partially blocking it. If you want the same flow exiting the hose that you had before stepping on it, you are going to have to increase the inflow. There is, therefore, going to be a great deal more pressure built up in the hose to accomplish that same flow rate however.

The bladder does just this--it increases its emptying pressure. It has no "sense" of the flow rate, but it does "read" pressure. In order to empty itself, higher and higher pressures are generated by working the muscles of the bladder harder and harder. Two things then occur. First, the muscles of the bladder thicken, called hypertrophy, much like a weightlifter's arms do. However, while this thickening allows the bladder to generate higher pressures to void, the muscles fail to completely relax when they're not at work, like Arnold Schwartzenegger's arms which fail to relax straight. This compromises the bladder's ability to hold as it can't stretch, and it leaves constant pressure in the bladder, which is interpreted in the brain as the need to urinate again. Thus, the bladder never feels as if it's empty.

Take some numbers in a relative sense, not as absolute. First when younger, our bladder rests say at a pressure of 15 centimeters of water pressure and holds this pressure over a wide volume of 300 to 400 milliliters (ml) as our bladder fills. When we urinate, the pressure may reach 30 centimeters or so. It's not unusual for the man with detrusor instability, that is, with this chronically high pressure in his bladder which as developed from chronic high pressure urinating, to have resting pressures of 30 to 40 centimeters and voiding pressures of 60 to 80 centimeters.

Second, as a result of the blockage and the need to work harder to urinate, the bladder tires before it can completely empty. This means that each time the gentleman urinates, he probably has a significant amount of urine left behind in the bladder. As with a balloon, if you don't let all of the air out, it will not take as many puffs to fill it again. Translated, the interval of time between each urination is lessened because the bladder is always at least half-full, for example.

Muscle thickening and incomplete emptying, taken together, can explain the significantly bothersome symptoms which the gentleman with BPH can experience. He's "crimped" at both ends, not only does he not empty his "balloon" (bladder) all the way, his "balloon" is often considerably smaller. Once, his bladder held 400 ml and he emptied that with a first notice of the need to void at 350 ml or so. Now, he holds 300 ml or so, empties to a residual of 100 ml (voids 200 ml at a time), meaning he's going twice as often to empty the same amount. Even at that, however, because of the high resting pressures in the bladder, he never does seem completely empty. Now throw in the fact that as we get older we progressively "house" more fluid in the soft tissues of our legs, which is taken back into the bloodstream and filtered off as urine by the kidneys by the elevation of our legs at night while in bed. In other words, even with fluid restrictions this gentleman may be up several times at night because in addition to having a smaller balloon which empties poorly, more "air" is being forced into it.

In Bladder Basics, Chapter 9, we discuss how the brain can look the other way through habituation or accommodation as to not be constantly distracted by the bladder's need to go. What happens then, however, is that when the bladder's message is ultimately interpreted as a serious need to urinate, it has already begun to do so. Translated into what the patient experiences is a sudden uncontrollable urge to void and some urge incontinence (leakage associated with the urge), frequently experienced upon awakening from sleep.

In some people, the muscles of the bladder may stretch to the point where they do not have good "purchase" upon each other with which to contract and empty. Think of this with the following example. Link the fingers of each hand with the tips of the fingers interlocking through their full length. They can pull tightly against each other. Now, place them interlocking only at their tips, without much purchase at all. In this arrangement, much like with the bladder filled to its capacity, the muscles will be able to squeeze only a portion of the contents out, leaving a significant amount left behind. Again, the balloon will be filled very rapidly as it never is emptied. Let's look at some numbers.

When younger, our patient was able to hold 400 ml, emptied 400 ml, and felt an urge to go at 350 ml or so. Now, over several years time, he can hold 800 ml, but when he urinates he only empties 200 ml at a time, leaving 600 ml behind, and not feeling the need to go until 790 ml when he better"get there in a hurry". He goes twice as often and only half as much. In the morning upon awakening especially and often through the day, he may have tremendous difficulty initiating the stream because during sleep he allowed those muscle fibers to stretch even more than he would normally during the day. They are pulling together from their very "fingertips". These patients also have the production of additional urine when the legs are elevated to accentuate the problem of incomplete emptying.

MEDICAL/SURGICAL INDICATIONS

If the prostate enlargement itself is not harmful, what are the indications to treat medically or to perform surgery to correct prostate obstruction of the urinary channel?

Bladder pressures, whether a result of high resting pressures from muscle thickening or the pressures generated from a tense, full, but thinned, bladder can, in their worst stages, result in kidney damage from blockage of the ureters, the tubes draining each kidney into the bladder. The tubes dilate or stretch, called hydronephrosis, resulting in poor filtration by the kidneys and kidney failure. This used to be seen quite frequently, but with more public awareness of prostate problems and less public tolerance for urinary disorders, this is encountered only occasionally. However, when encountered, the kidney function is most generally retrieved by placing a catheter in the bladder and careful fluid and electrolyte replenishment in an inpatient hospital setting. Once stabilized, the prostate is addressed surgically if the patient's overall medical status would allow surgery.

Occasionally, as a result of the residual urine which these patients continually carry, recurrent urinary tract infections become problematic. These may be hallmarked by foul urine and incontinence, caused as the infection results in irritability and further spasticity (contracting difficult to control) in an already hyperactive bladder. More importantly, infections which embed themselves in the substance of the prostate or ascend up the ureters to the kidneys can gain access into the bloodstream and develop urosepsis, an overwhelming infection which can have up to a 70% mortality. Infections then become an indication to perform prostate surgery.

On occasion, men with prostate hypertrophy may have gross (visible) hematuria, or blood in the urine. This results from voiding under such very high pressures that the blood vessels lining the bladder or prostate may rupture. The bleeding can be severe enough to require hospital admission, placement of a catheter to drain the bladder and to irrigate it free of clots,and even to transfuse the patient. A full urologic evaluation is required in these patients to assure that a tumor, i.e. a tumor of the kidney, is not overlooked in assuming that the bleeding is from the bladder or prostate. Bleeding is an indication to proceed with surgery.

Urinary retention, that is, the complete inability to urinate even perhaps without any bleeding or signs of kidney function compromise, is an indication to proceed with surgical intervention.

In the absence of any direct indications to proceed with surgical intervention, the decision to proceed with prostate surgery is truly that of the patient. If urinary habits begin to direct lifestyle to the point that they are "significantly" bothersome or distracting, then it's time to be treated. If, for instance, the patient loves to travel but is afraid to ride in an airplane or to drive any distance in a car because of the fear of wetting, then it's time to get it done. If he likes to play golf, but can only go up and down a fairway or two without finding a tree to hide behind, it's time. If he's crabby and grumpy all the time from never a getting a good night's sleep because of nocturia (nighttime urination), then it's time. The urologist will frequently suggest an outpatient evaluation to assess medically the severity of the problem and to assist the patient in placing his problems on the spectrum of all patient's with similar complaints, but the decision to proceed with medical or surgical intervention is a deeply personal one.

The American Urological Association (AUA) has developed a Symptom Index for BPH (See Figure 7-1). It is an attempt to place some objectivity to the more subjective complaints which we have discussed as mild (0 to 7), moderate (8 to 19), or severe (20 to 35). The use of this index is included in the AUA guidelines for the evaluation and treatment of BPH.

EVALUATION

The evaluation of the patient with BPH starts with a complete history and physical exam, including some assessment of a specific urinary symptom index (See Figure 7-1) and to assure that there are no factors from other systems or ailments which may be contributory. A routine check of the urine (urinalysis) will detect the chemical constituents of the urine suggesting any associated kidney problems, diabetes mellitus by the check of urinary sugar included, and for blood both chemically and by a look microscopically. Also, inflammatory or pus cells can be detected chemically and microscopically, indicating possible inflammation or infection. On occasion, bacteria, the organisms responsible for infection can even be seen. Blood tests, the BUN (blood urea nitrogen) and Cr. (short for creatinine), are routinely checked to assess good kidney function. These are mandatory if the IVP (intravenous pyelogram, an xray of the kidneys) is to be ordered by the urologist, to assure the contrast administered into the vein can be cleared readily from the system by the kidneys. The PSA (prostatic specific antigen) is ordered to rule-out any occult prostate malignancy.

The cystourethroscopy, or look in the bladder and prostate, remains useful in the evaluation particularly to detect other pathology which may be present, i.e. an otherwise undetected bladder carcinoma if hematuria (blood in the urine) is found on the routine urinalysis. Interestingly, although cystoscopy has been the gold standard evaluation used by urologists to assess the presence or absence of obstruction, recent guidelines from the federal government based upon studies performed utilize the Symptom Index and other parameters such as the flow rate and residual urine (See below). The cystoscopy, if indicated, can be accomplished either in the urologist's office or in the outpatient setting under a local anesthetic, i.e. a numbing gel is placed into the penis for 3 to 5 minutes after the genitalia have been sterilely prepped and draped. Many urologists use a flexible instrument for this evaluation which approximates the sensation of being catheterized. Used competently and gently, the rigid cystoscope is still tolerated very well.

Frequently, this will be teamed with some assessment of the patient's ability to empty the bladder by a uroflow and post-void residual. The patient is asked to void into a special toilet-like device which measures the rate at which the urine is passed, i.e. 5 ml per second, and the total amount voided, i.e. 400 ml. The patient is then catheterized, or if this study is performed prior to the cystoscopy, the cystoscope is passed and the residual urine, that left in the bladder at the completion of urination, is retrieved and measured. Generally speaking, any residual urine of 100 ml. or greater is significant. Flow rates of greater than 20 ml. per second are normal, between 10 ml. and 20 ml. per second and gray zone, and less than 10 ml. per second are indicative of a highly obstructed system.

AUA SYMPTOM INDEX FOR BPH

Not at all	Less than 1 time	Less than half the time	About half the time	More than half the time	Almost always
0	1	2	3	4	5

1. Over the past month, how often have you had a sensation of not emptying your bladder completely after you finished urinating? _____

2. Over the past month or so, how often have you had to urinate again less than two hours after you finished urinating? _____

3. Over the past month or so, how often have you found that you stopped and started again several times when you urinated? _____

4. Over the past month or so, how often have you found it difficult to postpone urination? _____

5. Over the past month or so, how often have you had a weak urinary stream? _____

6. Over the past month or so, how often have you had to push or strain to begin urination? _____

7. Over the last month, how many times did you most typically get up to urinate from the time you went to bed at night until the time you got up in the morning (0, 1 time...to 5 or more times)? _____

Total Symptom Score: _____

Figure 7-1: The AUA Symptom Index for BPH.

If associated medical conditions dictate, i.e. the gentleman has had a stroke, then a full urodynamic study is indicated to assess for a neurogenic bladder. The CMG (cystometrogram) is a measure of the pressures of the bladder as it is gently filled through a catheter and requires a piece of equipment which minimally may run $15,000. In conjunction with the CMG, another test called the EMG (electromyogram) is performed. This is performed by the placement of EKG pads, like those placed on your chest to perform the heart's tracing, on the buttocks to assess the smooth coordination of the working of the pelvic floor muscles with that of the bladder (See Bladder Basics, Chapter 9).

TREATMENT

The treatment of prostate enlargement falls into two categories: medical and surgical.

Generally, medical treatments can be expected to improve symptoms of blockage in milder cases. The mechanism of action is either a relaxation of the neck of the bladder or an actual shrinkage of the substance of the prostate. Carefully selected, improvements in symptoms of obstruction or bladder irritability from high pressure voiding can be seen in 25 to 60% of patients depending upon the study quoted.

Refer to Chapter 9, Bladder Basics: if one can relax the neck of the bladder, the pressures necessary to empty the bladder will be less and bladder emptying will be improved. Hytrin® (terazosin), Minipres® (prazosin), and Cardura® (doxazosin) all accomplish this successfully--each with decided advantages and disadvantages. Hytrin® is the only medication in this group with FDA approval for this "indication", although Minipres® and Cardura® are frequently utilized. By virtue of their mechanism of action each can lower the blood pressure, which may be good if the patient's is generally elevated, but it may cause some dizziness in the patient with generally normal to low pressure, at least when the medication is first started. In the sexually active patient, an inability to completely tighten the neck of the bladder during ejaculation may result in retrograde ejaculation, or ejaculation into the bladder. While all the sensations associated with orgasm are the same, little is jettisoned and a cloudiness or clumpiness in the urine is noted the first urination or two after orgasm. The effectiveness of long term use of these medications remains to be determined.

The second pharmacotherapy (medical) for BPH centers around the maintenance and growth of prostate volume as dependent upon dihydrotestosterone (DHT), a male hormone. At least 6 different drugs are at the disposal of the urologist for this form of treatment. However, with all side-effects considered, only one is a realistic candidate, namely, Proscar® (finasteride). Proscar® can be expected to achieve its result within 6 to 12 months. Taken once per day compliance should be reasonably good. Approximately 25 to 33% will see appreciable improvement in urinary flow rates.

While useful in the treatment of BPH, the selection of patients who might garner benefit is extremely important. Also important is the consideration of the ongoing need to continue the medication and the continued expense of its purchase.

Surgical treatments of BPH all eliminate, in one fashion or another, the central "fruit" portion of the prostate thereby removing the obstructing tissue and increasing the aperture through which the bladder must force the urine. Balloon dilation of the prostate works on the principle that a balloon place in the prostate by inflation will, when expanded, compress the surrounding ring of prostate tissue making the channel more open. While successful in the short term, this technique has a high failure rate by one year, making its use and the clinical indications very limited. One very useful scenario is the patient who might not be thought of as a good surgical candidate--perhaps having recently had another surgery or medical setback, i.e. a stroke. This patient may be rendered catheter-free by this procedure. He then can be returned for his definitive procedure, if necessary, in 6 months to a year when he is medically more able to withstand the surgical procedure.

Transurethral laser incision of the prostate (TULIP) is a technique wherein the prostate is incised or cut utilizing laser technology through the cystoscope passed through the penis. Think of this as cutting or incising a ring which will then spring open. Less invasive, this can frequently be performed in the outpatient setting and works very well for long term good results in patients whose prostates are more collar-type in configuration rather than large glandular type "fruity" prostates. TULIP has not achieved government approval as a recognized procedure, although it is widely utilized and successfully performed.

TUMP, transurethral microwave prostatectomy, is a technology on the horizon which employs the use of a microwave probe to treat the prostate causing it to "melt" as the cells die. Biopsies are done to ensure that no cancer of the prostate exists as no surgical specimen is available by the procedure. TUMP is under FDA study.

Laser prostatectomy, utilizing laser energy to destroy the obstructing prostate tissue (as opposed to the previously described incision of the prostate and bladder neck), is being utilized with increasing frequency. Because the tissue is destroyed rather than "cut out" as described in the TURP described below, most urologists perform needle biopsies with the procedure to provide tissue diagnosis to rule-out occult (unsuspected) cancer of the prostate.

The "gold standard" remains the transurethral resection of the prostate (TURP). The procedure is performed through a resectoscope (or large cystoscope) passed through the penis and involves trimming out the tissue from the inside, much like drilling a hole in the wall and making it larger and lager by coring it out from the center outward. The tissue is retrieved by a suction device from the bladder and a catheter is placed for a few days post operatively. The tissue is looked at by the pathologist to look for unsuspected cancer.

The hospital stay is usually 2 or 3 post-operative days total with a catheter in place for the first day or two usually. An additional 4 to 6 weeks of limitations post-operatively are required to ensure adequate healing. Think of the prostate after this surgery as a giant scrape. If you squeeze a scrape it bleeds; once covered with its new skin, you can squeeze a scrape all you want, and it won't bleed. During the time of limitations we're waiting for this new skin covering to complete its covering of the lining of the prostate. You squeeze the prostate by lifting, straining, grunting, even pushing too hard to have a vigorous bowel movement. Driving, in and of itself, is not vigorous, but invites other activities, i.e. lifting a sack of groceries into the trunk, which may be. In my own practice, I keep the gentlemans home for the first week post discharge, the second week he can be out with someone else driving and no vigorous activity, and during the third week he is not restricted except for no lifting or straining. Over the next two to three weeks, incremental levels of activity are approved, with normal activity levels achieved by approximately 6 weeks post-operatively. Sexual activity is probably OK at about 4 weeks.

At 7 years post procedure, approximately 50% of men are having symptoms once again of which one-half (or 25% of the original group) will go on to require a second procedure 7 to 10 years subsequent to their original procedures. However, with better medical treatments, a significant portion of theses men will respond to medical management as a majority of their prostate will have been addressed by their initial surgery.

As an aside, in the 6th decade (that is, of men in their 50's), 10 to 15% of men having this operation for seemingly benign disease will have at least a single area of cancer detected in their surgical specimen. The rate goes up by approximately 10% per decade. As our experience with the PSA grows, unsuspected cancer will probably occur less and less.

Approximately 10% of prostate surgery for benign conditions require open surgery, that is through an incision. This is for two reasons: first, the prostate is just too large to be done through the channel or scope; second, there is an associated condition which requires correction in the same surgical setting, i.e. a bladder stone formed as a result of residual urine crystallizing out into a stone which over time gradually enlarges to a point that it cannot be passed.

If the prostate cannot be safely resected through the resectoscope (a larger cystoscope through which the prostate can be chiseled out) in roughly one hour, then the procedure is scheduled through an incision. The procedure involves removing the central portion of the prostate much like removing the fruit portion an orange leaving the peel intact. In fact, the plane between the central adenoma to be removed and the surgical capsule which is like the peel and which remains behind intact in operations for BPH. In the radical prostatectomy, the surgery performed for cancer of the prostate both the peel and the fruit are removed intact. While the post-operative rehabilitation period may be longer than that for transurethral surgery, the overall long term results are superior because the entire adenoma is removed rather than a portion which is generally the case with even the best of resections. Addressing the associated pathology, i.e. the bladder stone or the bladder diverticulum (a pouch or hernia-like protrusion of the bladder as a result of high pressure voiding) may improve the overall clinical results as well.

In patients with chronic high pressure voiding and a resultant spastic bladder, better than 75% will see an improvement by alleviating the obstruction. In those who don't improve, a bladder relaxant can be used to relax the bladder to resolve the frequency and urgency (See Bladder Basics, Chapter 9).

While treatment options may in fact cause confusion for the patient, carefully selected and with reasonable expectations of the results, these patients can generally be afforded a marked improvement in lifestyle with, hopefully, few experiencing complications.

Additional imformation can be obtained by writing the Agency for Health Care Policy and Research (AHCPR) Publications Clearinghouse, P.O. Box 8547, Silver Spring, MD, 20907; or call toll free (800) 358-9295 and ask for AHCPR Publication No. 94-0584, *Treating Your Enlarged Prostate: Patient Guide.*

CHAPTER 8

PROSTATE CANCER

Cancer of the prostate.

Prostate cancer accounts for approximately 18 to 22 % of all cancers in men over the age of age 55. It is now the leading type of male cancer with greater than 32,000 deaths attributable to this disease and 122,000 new cases expected to be reported this year. Unfortunately, our historical batting average is that approximately one third of men present with disease already outside the prostate, and therefore are not curable by any of today's treatments. Despite the variety of therapeutic measures employed during the last sixty years, the age adjusted death rate has doubled in that time. The combination of factors including increased public awareness, improved blood testing, and improved technology each should increase our ability to detect the disease. Utilizing these new developments should allow us to more successfully treat prostate cancer, but this can only be accurately stated with time. Theses factors will each be discussed in this chapter.

Recent political figures, i.e. Senator Alan Cranston, Senator Robert Dole and high profile figures like Roone Arledge, the network executive, and Bill Bixby, have assisted in bringing prostate cancer to the forefront by virtue of making their disease public. Early detection is critically important and any assistance for getting to a physician for a rectal exam and consideration of bloodwork is helpful.

There is no substitute for an annual rectal exam in any man over the age of 40 to 45.

The detection of prostate cancer by rectal exam alone is 30%, however it cannot be excluded as a part of an examination. In addition to the examination of the prostate gland, the examination of the rectum itself for masses and the check of the stool for any evidence of blood for early detection of colon cancer is critically important in this age group as well. When taken in conjunction with the PSA (the prostatic specific antigen--a blood test) the detection rate increases to nearly 70%.

The PSA was developed as a means to improve upon our early detection of prostate cancer. Historically, the blood test used was the Acid Phosphatase. This test was widely employed and highly useful. However, it had approximately a 10% false positive and 10% false negative rate. In other words, the Acid Phosphatase was abnormal 10% of the time (worrisome for cancer) although the gentleman did not have prostate cancer (false positive). Conversely, 10% of the time the gentleman had prostate cancer even with a normal Acid Phosphatase (false negative). The PSA roughly halved the false negative (that is, only 5% of the time is the test negative with a gentleman with prostate cancer); however, it doubled to 20% the false positive (that is, the test is elevated and therefore worrisome for cancer). Of these two sides of the coin, the bigger sin is to never have suspected cancer by virtue of a normal blood test. The abnormal blood test in the patient found not to have cancer by additional evaluation does cause worry and expense, but does assure the absence of cancer when fully evaluated.

Because of the concern regarding the expense incurred as a result of additional testing, we are attempting to develop a spectrum of concern regarding the results of the PSA. The normal values in this are 0 to 4.0. Therefore, if your result is less than 4 and there is no suspicion on rectal exam of prostate cancer, your likelihood of having prostate cancer is well less than 5 %. The difficulty comes in the blood test which is "marginal".

In the range between 4 to 10, the additional testing must be tailored by several features--the individual patient's exam, other medical conditions, and temperament of the patient to "observing" an abnormal result. Let me explain, but let me first say that this represents one of the many"gray-zones" where one must practice the art of medicine--in other words, this in no way reflects dogma, varies between among urologists, and will change over time as we gain additional experience with the PSA and the assay changes.

With the patient whose result is between 4 and 10, the options are two:

      1) proceed to ultrasound and if there are areas of concern to biopsy (explained later); or
      2) sequential rectal exams (say, done quarterly) with sequential PSA's performed as well.

If the PSA remains unchanged or lowers without any change noted on the rectal exam, then continued observation is employed (i.e., after one year of quarterly checks, the frequency is reduced to twice yearly for two years, then annually). If, however, the PSA continues a trend upward then an ultrasound and biopsy would be indicated.

Any decision for continued observation is dependent upon the ability to perform a complete rectal exam which is unequivocally normal. If there is any concern regarding the "texture" of the prostate on rectal exam, or if the prostate is so large that it cannot be examined in its entirety, then ultrasound is a necessary adjunct.

Obviously there are gray-zones of the gray-zones. That is, observation in the gentleman with a PSA of 5 is more "comfortable" than in the gentleman whose value is 9.6. This is where you also must ask your patient how nervous he is going to be with a test result which is not totally normal. The age of the patient too may have a bearing on the course of action too. The potential delay is diagnosis may not affect outcome in the slightest in the 85 year-old man; conversely, not all the data is in, but urologists worry about the same time delay in the diagnosis of the 55 year old. The data seems to suggest that if the PSA's are closely monitored in a timely fashion and teamed with a good rectal exam, there will be ample "lead-time" afforded by change in the PSA to allow diagnosis by biopsy and intervention, i.e. surgery, without compromising the outcome for the patient.

One final note regarding the PSA. It is not a substitute for a rectal exam. If you were to poll practicing urologists, nearly, if not entirely, 100% would have had a case of a prostate lump to be biopsy-proven as cancer with a "normal" PSA. In other words, the two tools (a good rectal exam and the PSA) must be used to complement each other.

Enter the prostate ultrasound. This is a machine which shows us the architecture of the prostate by bouncing painless sound waves off of the gland in much the same way a submarine uses sonar to look at the topography of the ocean floor. A probe about the size of an average-sized thumb is placed in the rectum. The probe has a small water chamber at its end which is gently filled to allow a smooth interface between the probe and the gland. It's not a comfortable examination--but it's tolerable, easily accomplished with the patient awake and utilizing only a local anesthetic, i.e. xylocaine jelly place in the rectum. The study usually takes approximately 10 to 15 minutes. The prostate can be looked at in several different views and its size estimated by applying its length, width, and height into a calculation to estimate volume. The ultrasound study shows us any areas of concern and most ultrasound units come with a software option which will allow us to line up on the screen any areas of concern to direct the biopsy "gun", a spring-loaded needle which, when activated, obtains a small core of tissue to be looked at under the microscope. The prostate ultrasound shows the trajectory and anticipated "snatch" point of the biopsy. This allows us to biopsy with a very high degree of accuracy and because the action of the biopsy device is so quick, relatively with "tolerable" discomfort. The gentlemen wince, much like having blood drawn, but the discomfort is transient.

Preparation for the ultrasound and biopsy usually involves little more than a gentle enema shortly before the study and some antibiotic coverage, particularly if biopsies are to be obtained. If the gentleman is on blood thinners or chronic aspirin use, it is probably safer regarding risk of bleeding after the biopsy that these be discontinued prior and normalcy of clotting ability be assured by a check of clotting studies. However, in certain situations, the risk posed to the patient is so high in removing the blood thinners that we continue them even in light of the potential risk to cause bleeding by the biopsy itself.

The beauty of this technique is the accuracy with which it allows you to perform biopsies. Our fear is not the positive biopsy, because in that situation the diagnosis has been made, and while additional information will need to be obtained in the form of additional testing, treatment will be initiated for the prostate cancer shortly. The real advantage of this technique is the relative peace of mind for both the patient and the urologist in the biopsy which is negative--that is, the one which is not positive for cancer. A negative biopsy in the presence of cancer will delay diagnosis, thereby delaying treatment, and potentially affecting outcome for the patient. Biopsies done in this fashion are done with much greater accuracy.

The additional use of the ultrasound can be in obtaining "controlled random biopsies." In this setting, no discreet abnormalities are seen during the study and yet there remains a high suspicion for cancer, i.e. the PSA is extremely high. Mentally think of the prostate as heart-shaped and divide it into a right and left side. Biopsies are performed at the top, in the middle, and at the bottom of the gland yielding six (three on each side, right and left) well spaced specimens to hopefully reflect any cancer which may not be evident either to the examiners rectal examination or to the ultrasound technology itself.

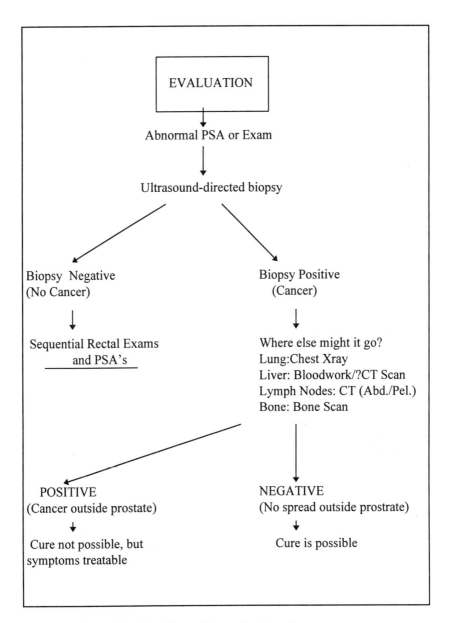

Figure 8-1: Algorithm of the evaluation of prostate cancer.
(Treatment is continued in Figure 8-5.)

One final use of the prostate ultrasound is the use of the measured volume as an index of suspicion for cancer. As the prostate enlarges, the PSA will go up as well. The two can be indexed against each other so that if the PSA goes up significantly more that what we would expect by the measured change in volume, we would be more worried about cancer in that setting.

Let's now change gears--much like many men have to do after going through the rectal exam, the PSA, and the ultrasound with a biopsy for the hypothetical finding of prostate cancer. Let's assume that the biopsy is positive for cancer.

The approach to prostate cancer is much the same as with cancer of any source in that there is a set of sequential questions to answer in order to best understand the extent of disease and to select the most effective treatment. These include:

       1.) What is the extent of my cancer in the organ of origin? (in our discussion, in the prostate.)
       2.) Where else does this cancer go, and is it there?
       3.) What are the treatment options for my disease?
       4.) What is the best treatment option?
       5.) What is the expected outcome?

Let's take these one at a time. I have found the easiest way to communicate this information to patients and family members is by the use of dendograms, or flow diagrams. This serves to give an overall sense of direction and at the same time answering one question at a time. Figure 8-1 is a sample diagram for prostate cancer which will be referred to in the subsequent discussion.

Following the dendogram: The ultrasound allows us to visualize the architecture of the prostate. Abnormal architecture is biopsied under direct visualization; that is, we can actually direct and watch the biopsy performed as it is taken from those areas of concern. We can therefore gain some sense of the extent of involvement by the appearance on ultrasound and also by the number of biopsies which are positive.

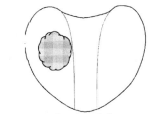

Figure 8-2: A prostate gland nodule.

Our example, Figure 8-2, above shows a 1 centimeter (just shy of ½ inch) nodule or lump in the left prostate which was positive for cancer by biopsy. If the biopsies were positive in areas 1 and 3 in addition to the nodule labeled 2, we would be able to counsel the patient that the disease is more extensive than that which is felt manually. With biopsies 4, 5, and 6 all negative we have the good news that the disease appears confined to ½ of the prostate. If we had demonstrated that the lump extended into the tissues next to, but definitely outside of the prostate (as depicted in Figure 8-3), this patient would be again counseled differently.

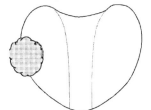

Figure 8-3: Prostate gland nodule extending outside the prostate gland.

The point to this discussion is that the ultrasound and the controlled random biopsies can give us a "sense" of the extent of disease within the prostate. However, there is debate as to the accuracy particularly in borderline cases.

The PSA is the first indicator of whether or not the disease is outside of the prostate. The PSA goes up directly related to the volume or size of disease. The larger the cancer, the more likely it is to have spread elsewhere. PSA's of greater than 20 in diagnosed prostate cancer are worrisome for spread elsewhere, and greater than 40 are extremely worrisome. As an aside, the PSA is also used in patients who are undergoing or who have completed treatment for prostate cancer as a means of detecting early recurrence or regrowth of cancer.

Prostate cancer goes to bone, particularly the bones of the pelvis and the lower spine (lumbosacral spine). A bone scan, which is a test in which a radioactive material is injected and collects in abnormal bones and joints, will be positive long before we see areas of concern on routine bone xrays. Interestingly, the total xray dose to which the patient is exposed is less than one chest xray for this entire scan--showing us all of the bones in the human body.

Prostate cancer goes to the lung and therefore a standard chest xray is included in the metastatic evaluation for these patients.

Prostate cancer may deposit into the liver by being spread through the bloodstream. The liver can be checked by blood tests included in a standard chemistry profile, thousands of which are ordered on a daily basis for a variety of reasons through doctors' offices. The liver can also be examined by use of an xray test called the CT Scan (or Cat Scanner). This enables us to see all of the internal organs and shows us very accurately any architectural abnormalities present.

Finally, the lymph nodes are filters--filtering cancer, infection, and other foreign matter and chemicals. When you were a child and had a sore throat, frequently you had tender lumps along your windpipe (trachea) or under your jawbone (mandible). These were inflamed lymph nodes doing their job of filtering infection and toxins, preventing them from being disseminated through out your body. The lymph nodes filtering the prostate sit deep within the pelvis. The large blood vessel which delivers the blood form the heart is called the aorta. It branches at approximately the umbilicus (belly button), sending a branch to each leg called the iliac artery (See Figure 8-4).

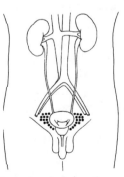

Figure 8-4: Lymph nodes draining the prostate gland.

The aorta pulsing is what you feel throbbing deep inside of you when you step off the curb prematurely and almost get run over by a bus. The branches are what you feel pulsing in each groin as the iliac artery descends from inside the abdomen to become the femoral artery as it enters the upper leg. The pocket between the iliac artery and the bladder and prostate (to each side) is called the obturator fossa and is the area where the lymph nodes draining the prostate and bladder reside. The lymph nodes from this area can be removed with little to no side-effects to check for spread. If the lymph nodes contain cancer, the disease is not curable but is treatable, medically. If the lymph nodes are negative for cancer (contain no cancer), then the disease is curable either by surgical removal of the gland or by radiation therapy (See Figure 8-5).

The decision to have radical cancer surgery for prostrate cancer or radiation therapy is a complex decision and one which is debated even among the "experts". The surgery itself is one of the most challenging to perform and is one which requires patience and tincture of time on the part of the patient from which to rebound. The surgery is generally performed at the same time as the lymph node dissection. If the nodes contain cancer (nodes positive), then no prostatectomy is performed. If the nodes are negative for cancer, the patient has consented to proceeding with the prostatectomy for curative surgery at the same surgical setting.

In essence, a radical prostatectomy involves the removal of the prostate in its entirety, the attached glands called the seminal vesicles, and a re-anastomosis (re-attaching) of the bladder to the urethra at the pelvic floor (See Figure 8-6). At the surgeon's discretion, the procedure can be performed in a manner termed "nerve-sparing", in which the nerves providing for erection are spared as they course near the prostate and urethra. While, potency-sparing is one of the most recent advances in the surgery for prostate cancer, no surgeon should compromise the cancer result in order to maintain potency . Erections can be maintained in approximately 60-70% of men who have good to excellent potency prior to the procedure.

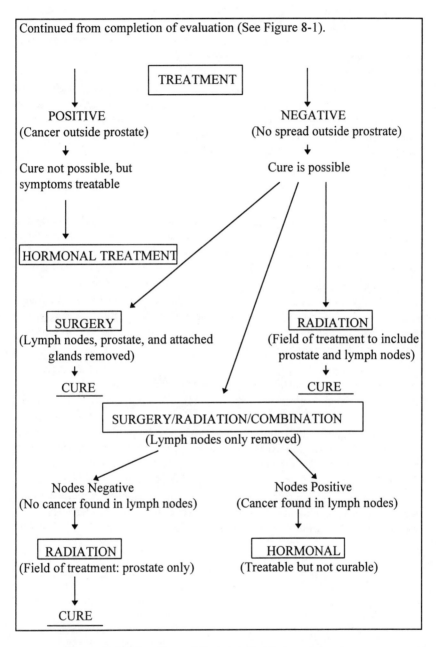

Figure 8-5: Algorithm of the treatment for prostate cancer.

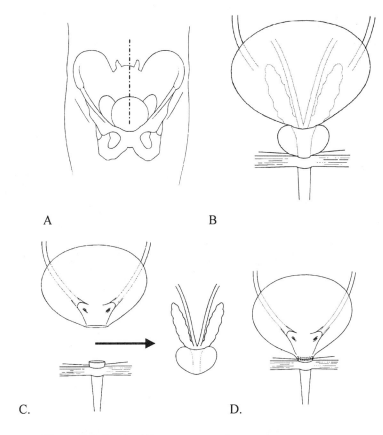

A   B

C.   D.

Figure 8-6: Radical Prostatectomy for prostate cancer.

Continence is maintained in 90% or better of men with newer techniques of excision and re-anastomosis, but this too is dependent upon the muscle tone prior to the procedure. The operation virtually eliminates 2 of the 3 mechanisms which provide dryness. To allow adequate healing, a catheter is left in place generally around 3 weeks post-operatively. Following its removal, it may take up to several weeks for complete confidence in urinary control to be regained. All of theses are easily overcome obstacles, but one for which the patient must be thoroughly counseled before proceeding.

Here's the $25 question: Is radical prostatectomy indicated in all patients with potentially curable cancer of the prostate (that is, those who, based only upon their extent of disease, are potentially curable)? Many will not be surgical candidates simply on the basis of other medical problems, i.e. prohibitive heart disease. Others will not be candidates simply because its thought that the disease will never give the problems, i.e. the 89 year old who is likely to die a death of another cause long before prostate cancer manifests with problems. (Unless his 125 year-old dad brought him in for the evaluation in the first place!) Others will simply not select surgery because they do not want any surgery. But how should the patient be counseled who is open to any option of treatment and whose disease presents as potentially curable?

This decision can be among the most difficult in life to make. Studies of conservative therapy (no treatment) of men with localized prostate cancer have demonstrated 75% will develop progression and 13 to 20% will die of their disease during the first 10 years after diagnosis. Clearly treatment is indicated, particularly if life expectancy is greater than one decade. The choice of treatment becomes almost a philosophical one because to choose a treatment for cure of prostate cancer, one must look at 12 to 15 years down the line before one sees appreciable differences in "cancer-free survival" between radiation and radical surgery. The reported 15-year disease-specific survival for men with localized prostate cancer following radical prostatectomy is 86% which compares favorably to 64% following external beam radiation. Therefore, many will say "Keep me going, don't set me back; I'll deal with 15 years from now if I get there." Others will assume they'll be there and say, "Let's cure this NOW! I never want to have to face this again." Who can argue with either answer--it's deeply personal and much the same in its formulation as any long-term commitment in the senior years. Generally speaking though, if the patient's age is under 70 and the overall health is good, radical prostatectomy is the most logical option for cure. Radiation therapy, however, is a very reasonable alternative as well, especially as the age approaches 70. Over 70, most would agree that radiation therapy to the prostate should be considered primary.

Radiation therapy is not without complications and inconveniences. Many patients experience various degrees of bowel and bladder irritation. Impotence up to 40 to 50% is reported as well. And once radiation therapy is administered, there can be no further radiation to the treated area should there be a cancer recurrence. Operating upon the prostate gland after it has been irradiated can be extremely difficult, sometimes impossible, with much higher rates of incontinence and other problems such as breakdown of the rectum leading to a communication between the bladder and the bowel which may require permanent colostomy. Cost is also a consideration. Radiation therapy costs can often approximate that of incurred surgical costs.

In my own practice, I have encouraged patients to have the status of the nodes evaluated before they receive radiation therapy. Particularly in sizable tumors on rectal exam, tumors which are more angry appearance under the microscope (moderately to poorly differentiated tumors), or patients with concerning elevation of the PSA (greater than 30 ng/ml), these can have up to a 20 to 30% chance of having cancer in the lymph nodes. If this is not discovered, radiation therapy will not cure them, and they will have gone through the treatments without benefit. In very mild appearing tumors (well-differentiated), low to normal PSA values, and/or a very small volume disease, i.e. not appreciable by rectal exam, there is less than a 5 % chance of positive lymph nodes, and therefore their removal for staging is probably of low yield. The lymph nodes can be removed through a a standard surgical procedure or by laparoscopic techniques. If patients are thought not to be surgical or laparoscopic candidates, or wish to proceed to radiation therapy without the benefit of lymph node staging, then the field of irradiation is widened to include the lymph node beds, perchance low volume cancer in the nodes could be potentially cured. This has never been substantiated. If the nodes have been removed and are negative for cancer, the field of radiation is only to the prostate.

Laparoscopy allows the nodes to be removed through special scopes thus eliminating a large incision with additional recuperative and disability time. The procedure generally is slightly longer (depending upon the individual urologist's experience level) and requires a general anesthetic as opposed to a regional (spinal) anesthetic which can be utilized for the incisional surgery. In the traditional incisional technique, the lower border of the belly cavity (peritoneal cavity) is pushed aside and never violated in order to remove the lymph nodes. With the laparoscopic technique, the peritoneal cavity is traversed to get to the nodes, thus a regional anesthetic could not keep the patient comfortable. While the complications are low for both, the laparoscopic technique is not without complication, i.e. the development of cyst collections called lymphocoeles, and the data is not entirely in on any potential additional risk for spillage of tumor into the belly cavity in those patients whose nodes are positive for cancer. Newer developments involve an approach which completely avoid entry into the belly cavity.

In summary then, if the lymph nodes are negative for cancer, locally applied treatment, either surgery or radiation can be curative. If the lymph nodes are positive, historical studies show us that either of these treatment regimens will not benefit the patient, as there are probably deposits of prostate cancer which are out of these fields of treatment which were not detected in the testing. Therefore, any treatment rendered will not be curative, and any administered, i.e. medications, will require distribution through the entire body to reach those areas which are destined to be sites of metastasis.

Treatment for prostate cancer which has left the confines of the prostate, and therefore is not thought to be curable, is based upon the premise that early on, a substantial portion of the prostate cancer cells are stimulated to grow by the male hormone, testosterone. Anything which prevents this stimulation will kill a predominant portion of the prostate cancer cells. Note I did not say kill all the prostate cancer cells. The reason is that prostate cancer, like all cancers, is a population of cells which share likenesses and have differences-- just like us. We're all human beings, yet we all have strengths and weaknesses. Eventually, after most or all of the "hormonally dependent" cancer cells have been eliminated, the hormonally independent cell lines will continue to grow and multiply and eventually, given enough time, consume the patient. Treatment is rendered because the patient is having problems, i.e. bone pain in a rib or shoulder because a deposit of prostate cancer is there and causing inflammation. Treatment can also be rendered in the asymptomatic patient because it's felt that this may lengthen the time through which they continue to remain without symptoms (called the clinical disease-free interval), although the eventual outcome, that is, death from prostate cancer is neither prevented or delayed. In other words, we may have helped the patient to feel better longer. Studies indicate that younger patients with high-grade (angry) tumors seem to derive the greatest benefit from this approach.

Hormonal treatment can be in the form of removal of the testicles surgically (which produce approximately 95% of testosterone-like compounds), tablets called D.E.S., an estrogen which shuts off the testicles' production of testosterone but have a high risk of blood clots, or injection compounds taken monthly, i.e. LUPRON® or ZOLADEX®, which do the same thing without the risk of blood clots. Some physicians team the injections with a medication taken orally called Eulexin® (flutamide), which completes the hormonal blockade. The success of Eulexin® (flutamide) in significantly altering clinical progress remains debatable. The cost of these mediations over the course of a patient's disease can be staggering. Removal of the testicles remains the most definitive and probably lowest cost of treatment. Medical management for medications alone may range between $450-

600/month. Given our government's heavy involvement in health care spending and the diagnosis and treatment of prostate cancer alone in this country has been estimated as high as $12 billion, we certainly will see changes mandated in the care of the patient with prostate cancer.

Once prostate cancer has become unresponsive to hormonal manipulation, the overall survival becomes poor, in the range of 9 to 18 months. While many chemotherapeutic agents have been investigated, the results have been exceedingly disappointing. SURAMIN®, which actor Bill Bixby reportedly received, is currently the most promising and is under investigation at a number of institutions across the country.

As with most malignancies, the key to cure is early detection. Prostate cancer is best detected early in "routine" medical care with a conscientiously performed rectal exam in conjunction with the performance of the PSA blood test. Insist on these certainly if you are 50 or older, or if you're 40 or older and your family history includes prostate cancer or you have been vasectomized 15 to 20 years or longer.

For further information write to the local chapter of the American Cancer Society for materials and activities in your area for prostate cancer. The Prostate Cancer Support Group International Newsletter entitled *Us Too* can be subscribed to by writing: 11211 N. 84th St., Scottsdale, AZ., 85260-6554 or by calling (602) 991-0821.

CHAPTER 9

BLADDER BASICS AND INCONTINENCE

Bladder function and causes of urine leakage.

Before one can understand urinary incontinence (leakage), one must have an understanding of the normal voiding cycle. There literally is a cycle, or repeated circle of activity, which is necessary to achieve socially acceptable urinary habits. The cycle has just two phases (See Figure 9-1). The first phase is the storage phase. Urine which is continually being made by the kidneys and presented to the bladder at a rate of between 2 to 10 ml. per minute (5 ml. per teaspoon) must be stored until a socially accepted opportunity occurs for its elimination. The bladder, which is literally a hollow muscle, serves as a reservoir to retain the urine.

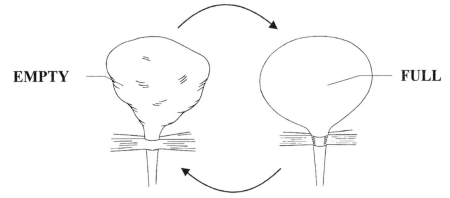

EMPTY   **FULL**

Figure 9-1: The voiding cycle.

The second phase of the voiding cycle is the emptying phase. Simply stated, this is the activity involved in the emptying of the reservoir. In actuality however, emptying completely is far more complex than it would first appear. To understand better both phases of the voiding cycle, we must broaden our understanding of the lower urinary tract anatomy and function.

The most important organ for continence is the bladder. It is made almost entirely of muscle with a hollow center and a special skin lining which is a different type of "skin" than that which covers us externally (See Chapter 14, Bladder Cancer and Blood in the Urine). The muscle, too, is different than that which we have in our arms or legs, for instance. It is called smooth muscle, and rather than being sudden and sporadic in its activity (like the sudden movement of my fingers as I type this text), it is more deliberate and smooth in its motion (like a worm moves with deliberate, smooth motion across the soil). The bladder and the intestine share a similarity in both have smooth-muscled walls. Differing in the arrangement of the muscle fibers, they nonetheless are the same type of muscle with similar innervation (nerve supply) and similar responses to medications. We'll discuss this last point a bit more later.

In addition to the bladder, the reservoir, we have a valve-type set-up to turn off and on the flow. Sphincters are such valves. They are circularly arranged muscles that when contracted close the valve or aperture and when relaxed open the valve or aperture allowing flow. We are blessed in the urinary tract with two valves to control the flow of urine.

The main valve or sphincter is fabricated from the pelvic floor muscles. The pelvic bones are fairly complex in their arrangement--made even more complex by the need to relate to the spine on the back side and to two legs at the hips on the down side. In a general sense however, you can understand them if you think of the pelvis as a ring. The muscles of the "floor" of the pelvis are like a piece of cloth stretched across this ring.

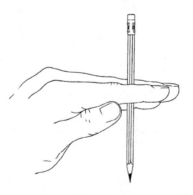

Figure 9-2: Analogy for the pelvic floor muscles.

To assist in better understanding how this sheet of muscle keeps you dry, place your hand stretched with all your fingers and thumb together and straight (See Figure 9-2). Now place a pencil between your ring and middle finger close to your hand. As long as you gently squeeze the pencil, it does not drop or slip. Relax your hand and it falls or slips out. So it is with our external sphincter. It squeezes our urethra, the tube which conducts the urine from the bladder to the outside,as it passes through the floor of the pelvis. When the muscle relaxes, the urine is freed to escape. In the continent (dry) patient, an increase in pressure with abdominal straining is simultaneously matched by a greater closure pressure of the urethra provided by the firm and minimally mobile pelvic floor. Interestingly the muscles in this sheet are of the same type as those of our arms and legs, called striated muscles. Its function is set up a little differently however. While most striated muscles are at rest until called upon to work, these muscles of the pelvic floor work all of the time until called to rest (to allow urination).

A second sphincter exists as well to assist in our urinary dryness. To explain this mechanism think back to when you were a kid and played with a "Chinese Finger Trap". Recall that as you placed your finger into each end of the spirally woven tube and pulled, the tube became tighter. Now think of the bladder as tear-shaped. The muscle fibers wrap in a spiral fashion around the neck of the bladder surrounding the urethra as it begins its descent to the outside (See Figure 9-3). Dryness is afforded by virtue of the muscles pulling

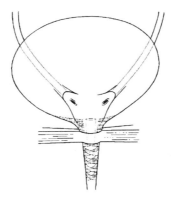

Figure 9-3: The bladder neck as a Chinese finger trap.

the tube tightly closed. To urinate, the nerves signal the relaxation of these fibers with the neck of the bladder and first part of the urethra opening to allow flow.

These two sphincters, the pelvic floor muscles and the bladder neck muscles, work in a coordinated fashion to assure dryness. You now have been given approximately 90% of what you need to know in order to understand any cause of incontinence. Also because of the similarity in the function and interaction of the smooth-muscled intestines and the rectum's passage through the pelvic floor musculature, you should have a fair understanding of the causes of fecal leakage as well.

Before we leave this discussion we should address one final concept which should help us summarize what we've accomplished thus far. The concept is called synergy; that is, two working together accomplish a greater result than the simple addition of each individually. In other words, with synergy 1+1 is greater than 2. Two people working on a project are frequently able to accomplish more than the simple additive effects of their efforts. The bladder and the sphincters working in a coordinated fashion are able to accomplish greater success in the storage and appropriately-timed emptying of urine than either individually.

The synergy of the bladder and sphincters can be summarized very simply:

With filling, the bladder relaxes and the sphincters contract.
With emptying, the bladder contracts and the sphincters relax.

Any failure in the coordination results in either suboptimal filling or inadequate emptying, either of which may render the person incontinent. We term this dyssynergy, or dyssynerrgia (dys=bad, synergy).

An example may serve to clarify this concept. Frequently, young children may have accidents because of "Busy Little Girl(Boy) Syndrome". This is a form of dyssynergy in which to keep from wetting the child has learned, perhaps overlearned, to keep the external sphincter tightened to finish their task at hand, i.e. watching television until the program is over or finishing play activity. We all do this from time to time. These children do this, however, almost every time they feel the need to urinate and over time it is so well learned that it becomes totally unconscious. What's so bad about this? What occurs is that during attempts to urinate the sphincter fails to relax as the bladder contracts--the coordinated effort is disrupted. Only a small portion of the bladder capacity is emptied, and therefore it will fill more rapidly to where the need to urinate again is sensed--like the balloon which is filled more rapidly when only a small amount of air is taken out than when it is emptied entirely. Because more pressure is needed by the bladder to force the urine out against the closed outlet, the child will be prone to more accidents because the pressure is sensed as urgency, a last-second notice that it is once again time to urinate. A third cause of incontinence from this learned behavior is a predisposition to infection because the bladder is never completely emptied. Any body fluid, whether in the bladder, intestine, lung, anywhere which is not turned over or drained completely and regularly can cause infection. Infection causes irritation, and irritation in an already irritated bladder is likely to yield incontinence.

The bladder's lining has sensory nerves just like those of the skin. They line the entire bladder but are more concentrated near the neck of the bladder in an area called the trigone (See Figure 9-3). As the word root "tri" suggests this is a triangular area, the three points of which are the two ureteral orifices (the holes of the tubular structure called the ureter which conducts the urine down from each kidney) and the funnel of the bladder neck to the urethra (the tube which conducts the urine to the outside). The brain really only hears one message from the bladder, "I've got to go!" As such, it is unable to decipher that a particular portion of the bladder is having trouble. The significance of this is that many conditions of the bladder, whether it be from infection, cancer, passage of a stone, or prostatitis, can all manifest with an irritable bladder because of any inflammation of the trigone. Each of these is discussed in its particular chapter.

Additionally, similar to intestinal problems which present with a generalized abdominal pain rather than an exact point of tenderness, bladder "pain" is occasionally difficult to " read" for the patient occasionally presenting with low back pain, pressure or pain in the low abdomen, vaginal complaints in females, and occasionally tenderness in the penis of males or the urethral meatus (opening through which we urinate) in both males and females.

Two additional anatomy considerations will round out our understanding of urine control. Angles play a very important part in the optimal function of certain anatomy. One very obvious example of this is the angle with which the thigh bone (femur) attaches at the hip, allowing full, painless range of motion. Another example is the bending of the last portion of the colon (large intestine) before it exits through the pelvic floor at the anus. These two bends prevent a full column of stool (feces) from pushing against the anus and leaking out. With the urinary system, the angle of the bladder as it attaches to the urethra is a very important supplement to support and position thereby resisting flow of urine out of the bladder, particularly in females. This will be discussed more fully in the Chapter 10, Stress Incontinence (leakage with lifting, straining, or laughing). This angle is such that it will assist in preventing leakage, and with urination or emptying it is changed to allow the swift exit of urine. It is the loss of this angle by a "hypermobile" urethra which results in abdominal pressure being converted into motion of the urethra and resultant urine loss in stress incontinence. As with the Chinese finger trap, to loosen it one pushes the fingers entrapped together and it gets shorter and wider allowing the fingers to be removed; as the urethra shortens and becomes wider with pelvic muscle weakening, it becomes unable to sustain dryness. Stated with another analogy, the urethra "accordians", losing its angulation, becoming shorter, and becoming wider--all of which contribute to wetness.

As an aside, if there is little to no salvageable anatomic support for continence (dryness), two options of treatment are at the urologist's disposal. First, an artificial sphincter (a prosthetic device) can be considered as a substitute (See Figure 9-4). These are positioned to wrap around the bladder

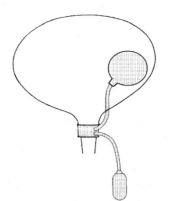

Figure 9-4: The prosthetic sphincter for urinary continence.

neck in females or the bladder neck or urethra in males and work by the inflatable portion gently constricting the enveloped tissues to attain dryness. With urination, the pump, which is situated in the labia of the female or the scrotum in the male, is pumped to suck the fluid out of the collar to be placed into a reservoir which is positioned in front of the bladder. A timed release valve then allows the collar to refill, and continence is resumed. Second, the patient's own tissues which envelop muscles (usually the abdominal muscle called the rectus abdominis), called fascia, can be harvested as a strip of tissue which then can be positioned at the neck of the bladder and positioned like a sling, hence the name "Sling Procedure".

The last concept to have all the pieces of the continence puzzle is actually a discussion of the nervous system (brain and nerves) and how it interacts with the bladder and sphincters which we've previously discussed. While this control is fairly complex, it can be understood as having two major parts. A reflex arc involves a muscle which must contract (the bladder), a nerve for sending sensory information back to the brain ("Hey! I'm full!"), and a motor nerve to carry the electrical message to fire the muscle ("OK, Go ahead.") (See Figure 9-5). Myriads of these reflex arcs control our bladders, the pelvic

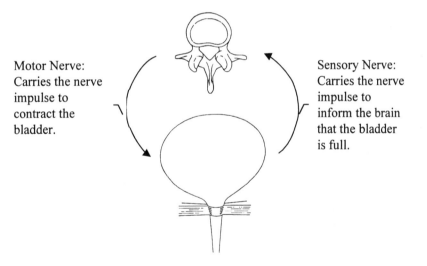

Motor Nerve: Carries the nerve impulse to contract the bladder.

Sensory Nerve: Carries the nerve impulse to inform the brain that the bladder is full.

Figure 9-5: The reflex arc with a sensory and motor nerve.

floor muscles, and all of our muscles for that matter. The arc tends to want to fire on its own--we see this as spasticity of an arm or leg, for example in the stroke victim. The reflex arc is constructed at the level of the spinal cord by the sensory nerve returning and the motor nerve exiting. The job of the spinal cord above that level and the brain is to dampen this independent activity of the reflex arc until the appropriate time to fire. When this control to coordinate is diminished or lost, we may see a spectrum of incontinence problems ranging from forms of dyssynergy to total spasticity of the bladder. Thus, in our previous example of the stroke patient, there has been a loss of the ability of the brain because of its injury to completely dampen the spontaneous firing of the reflex arcs. The bladder contracts whenever it wishes and incontinence occurs.

Another common neurologic problem with urinary incontinence is Multiple Sclerosis (M.S.). In fact, urinary symptoms may be the initial complaint in up to 15% of M.S. patients. With M.S., changes in the nerves within the spinal cord do not allow the conduction of electrical impulses up and down with their usual velocity. There may be hold-ups or detours. Orders, which are sent out by the brain to be received, interpreted, and implemented in a very timely and coordinated fashion, may not reach their destination on time. The coordinated control of the bladder and pelvic floor muscles, the synergy is disrupted. For example, the message "Relax!" is received by the external sphincter after the the bladder has already received and carried out its command, "Contract!".

With the information you've digested in this chapter, you now have the tools available to understand almost any form of incontinence. Incontinence in various forms and to varying degrees afflicts approximately 10 million Americans according to the United States Public Health Service, costing nearly $10 billion annually in health spending and lost productivity. Nearly 6 million sufferers have never sought treatment despite the fact that a majority of them could be cured with exercise or medications. Half of the nation's 1.5 million nursing home patients suffer from incontinence adding significantly to other health problems and costs.

For more information write or call: The Public Health Service for a free pamphlet, *Urinary Incontinence in Adults*, at (800) 358-9295 or (301) 495-3453 or by writing to the Agency for Health Care Policy and Research, Publications Clearinghouse, P.O. Box 8547, Silver Spring, MD. 20907. Information and support also can be obtained by writing to the Simon Foundation, P.O. Box 835, Wilmette, IL, 60091; or call (800) 23-SIMON for patient information or (708) 864-3913 for Headquarters; also, Help for Incontinent People (HIP), P.O. Box 544, Union, SC. 29379; (803) 579-7900 or (800) BLADDER.

CHAPTER 10

STRESS URINARY INCONTINENCE

Urine leakage with coughing, lifting, or straining.

One of the most devastating disorders which urologists treat in an otherwise healthy, active, many times young female is the condition wherein urinary leakage occurs with any type of straining activity--lifting, turning, exercising, coughing, even laughing. The devastation of this disorder can psychologically prove very disruptive to normal daily functioning of an otherwise healthy woman. Fortunately conditions such as this have "come out of the closet", and more women are seeking treatment. Seldom is there the need to resort to frequent changes of clothing, avoid social activities, or use inordinate amounts of padding.

Generally this type of incontinence occurs after multiple childbirths. The classic story is the woman at or around the time of her menopause who has had progressive leakage associated with straining type of activities and who has had at least 2 or 3 children. The spectrum of the amount of incontinence is varied--some women are totally intolerant of even the need to wear one pad per day, others seem not to mind using several pads per day. Many can be helped with the use of medication alone, others will need to resort to one of several surgical repairs.

The principles of bladder function and continence (dryness) were discussed in detail in Chapter 9, Bladder Basics. In brief summary, we discussed the bladder as a hollow muscle which must relax to hold urine, contract to empty itself, and work in coordination with two different types of valves or sphincters. We also discussed the importance of an intact nervous system coordinating all this activity, and finally--and most pertinent to this discussion--we touched upon the immobility of the urethra relative to the pelvic muscle floor in assisting in the maintaining of continence and the importance of urethral length and angles (position and support) between the bladder and the urethra (tube connecting the bladder to the outside). Before reading further, if there is confusion with what keeps us dry, reread Chapter 9.

The approach to stress urinary incontinence is one of first assuring ourselves as the physician and the patient that there are no other factors which might contribute to the anatomy problem rendering the patient to leak. It's as if we need to look to other factors first and then if nothing else is found except for the anatomy problem, attack that problem. Two examples may serve to illustrate this approach.

CASE STUDIES

Case One: Sharon is a 47 year old, active, 5th grade teacher. She has no medical problems. She has had no complicating surgeries (she's had only a gall bladder removal 10 years ago), and she has three children, all delivered vaginally, the youngest of which is 14 years old. She notes a bothersome leakage associated with activity, staining 2 to 3 inches of wetness daily on a pad she wears for protection and changes at lunch time. Interestingly, she's not wet on the weekends. An evaluation performed as an outpatient (which we will describe shortly) all proves to be normal, with the exception that her bladder is noted to be very generous in its size and that while her anatomy is not that of a 20 year old, her support should be capable of keeping her dry. What's the cause of Sharon's wetness?

Because of the nature of her work, Sharon probably does not void (urinate) with any regularity while working. She fills to her generous capacity and because of her beginnings of anatomy weakness of the pelvic floor she leaks when she's full and performs any activities which would increase the pressure in the bladder. Sharon does not need surgery. She needs to empty her bladder on a timed basis, say every 2 hours (like she does at home on the weekends), keeping it soft and supple so that when she does get down on the floor with a group of her 5th graders, the force exerted on the bladder can be absorbed rather than challenging the weakened sphincters attempting to keep her dry. She also may perform the Kegel exercises taught for many years by the gynecologists to re-assemble pelvic tone. Additionally, if these measures are less than satisfactory in results, Sharon may take medication which has an alpha-adrenergic effect to tighten the neck of the bladder. This is a common component in many cold and sinus preparations making it understandable why some folks experience difficulty urinating while taking cold preparations. These should not be taken on a daily basis because they will lose their effectiveness (called tachyphylaxis) and also have a side effect of elevating blood pressure in some patients. A dose around social need, i.e. a night out with friends with laughing and carrying on, can be quite successful in eliminating a socially embarrassing situation. Sharon is doing well taking

80

her "bathroom break" at 10 A.M. and 2 P.M. with her class and of course her noon break with lunch. On weekends, especially when she and her husband Brian go antique hunting, she takes an Entex LA® to have the assurance that she will not leak. She's been dry, without surgery, for nearly a year.

Case Two: Marcella represents a totally different type of incontinence problem. Now in her late 40's, she was divorced at 25. She never had children. Five years ago she was diagnosed as having cervical cancer (a type of cancer of the uterus) and was treated with radiation. She has gradually developed a severe leakage problem. Marcella notes that she gets very "short notice" when it's time to urinate.

She watches herself carefully, emptying regularly and watching what she drinks--"Caffeine drives my bladder wild!". It's not too much of a problem in the workplace. Her desk has been conveniently situated nearest the women's restroom. Marcella leaks profusely when she does anything strenuous, but, unlike Sharon who does not feel her bladder per say but only the wetness, Marcella's bladder lets her know it's going to empty and immediately does so and cannot be stopped. What's Marcella's problem?

An evaluation showed Marcella to have a small, shrunken bladder size from the radiation. Her pelvic muscles, muscles of the neck of the bladder, and the angles were all good. Because of the irritation and long-term effects upon the bladder by the radiation, Marcella's bladder at rest had two to three times the normal pressure in it . With increased pressure pushing on the outside of the bladder during activity, the brain could no longer ignore or control the bladder's desire to contract and empty itself. What can be done to help Marcella?

She has been improved, although not cured, with the use of bladder relaxants.

Marcella represents a group of patients which can be among the toughest to help. In extreme cases, surgery called "bladder augmentation" can be done to provide extra capacity. Pieces of intestine are attached to the bladder to add volume. Milder cases can be managed with bladder relaxants alone or in combination with medications to tighten the sphincters.

These two examples, Sharon's big bladder and Marcella's small bladder-- both with incontinence-- demonstrate that the perceived problem of wetness may occur with bladders of opposite types, or anywhere in between. What this necessitates then is a complete evaluation to avoid misdiagnosis, mistreatment (including misdirected surgery), and to avoid delay in accomplishing dryness. What is involved in the evaluation?

EVALUATION

Obviously, the first step is a complete history and physical examination to be sure that there are no contributing factors outside a primary anatomical problem, i.e. medications, prior surgeries, or symptoms which may be manifestations of a non-urologic cause of the problem (for instance a nervous system disorder, recurrent infection problem, endocrine problem like diabetes mellitus, or a primary gynecologic condition).

If the problem is assumed to be primarily with the urinary tract, infection can be ruled out by performing a urinalysis and urine for culture and sensitivity. The measurement of the bladder's capacity and ability to empty can be assessed by asking the patient to urinate into a receptacle, measuring its volume, and then catheterizing the patient in a sterile fashion to measure the residual urine (that is, the volume of urine left behind in the bladder upon completion of urination). Typically, a healthy bladder should empty itself to dryness. Realistically, it is not unusual to measure residuals of up to 100 ml. without too much concern in the adult female. Large residuals, i.e. 200-500 ml. may reflect a primary bladder problem or blockage problem preventing emptying that, if corrected, would allow even marginal anti-incontinence support to maintain dryness. For example, it is not unusual to find very generous bladder capacities in a diabetic with marked stress incontinence. If emptying can be improved by behavior modification techniques (i.e. timed-double voiding in which one voids every 3 to 4 hours by the clock rather than by need and returns to void approximately 20 to 30 minutes later for a second more complete emptying) then in many cases the stress maneuvering will be withstood without leakage because the bladder is not taut with no place to displace the pressure except by leakage.

"Formal" evaluation involves urodynamics, a more complex study of bladder functioning. This is a study done through a catheter placed into the bladder. The bladder is catheterized and gently and filled with either carbon dioxide or water while the pressures in the bladder are monitored and recorded in a tracing. More accurate determinations are done by measuring the pelvic floor muscle activity simultaneously through the use of EMG (electromyographic) equipment. This simply involves the placement of EKG patches (the type used to monitor the heart) on the buttocks. Below is an example of a normal tracing (See Figure 10-1).

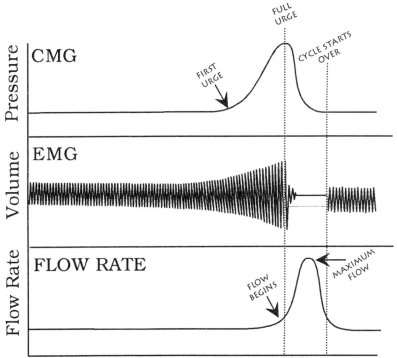

Figure 10-1: A normal urodynamic study.

Note that the bladder can maintain a relatively low pressure over a wide range of volume until its capacity is challenged and pressures rise. As the pressures increase, the muscle activity in the pelvic floor also increases and the muscles naturally work harder to maintain continence. Then, as the bladder empties, the pressure in the bladder falls and the pelvic muscle activity quiets to allow emptying. Concomitantly, the flow rate increases to a maximum, then falls as we approach the completion of urination. The bladder then once again relaxes, and the pelvic floor muscles again"kick in" to maintain continence as the bladder fills.

Many different aberrations may yield incontinence, but for the most part women with straightforward stress incontinence will have relatively normal urodynamics study. Marcella had a hypertonic (high-toned) bladder. Studies have shown though that a significant percentage, nearly one-third, of incontinent women will have a "mixed" stress and urge incontinence. This means that the leakage which they experience is not only from an anatomic problem but also from involuntary contraction of the bladder. This "instability" of the bladder results in continued leakage in a significant percentage (up to 20%) of those who fail surgical correction. Most of these will be assisted, though not totally cured, through the use of bladder relaxants.

A thorough history, complete physical examination including a Marshall Test performed with the pelvic examination, and the "Q-Tip®" Test provide the most meaningful information of the simple evaluation steps. In the Marshall Test, the patient is asked to strain both on her back and then in the upright position with the bladder moderately full. Stress incontinence shown should be corrected by elevating the neck of the bladder to either side of the urethra by the examiners fingers positioned at those points, thus mimicking the surgical correction. With the Q-Tip® Test, a Q-Tip® is positioned within the urethra and the swing of the Q-Tip® as the patient strains, in addition to the degree of leakage seen, displays the mobility of the urethra accounting for the leakage.

More sophisticated testing includes straining cystography (in which x-rays of the bladder and urethra are taken as the patient strains) and video/fluoro urodynamics (in which x-rays and pressure tests are performed simultaneously.

Interestingly, cystourethroscopy, or the examination of the bladder and urethra (tube connecting the bladder to the outside), historically has been the definitive test to delineate the anatomy. Typically it is done with a topical anesthetic agent and may be done with either a rigid or flexible instrument. This allows an examination of the interior of the bladder to visually assess size, contour, the presence/absence of other problems, and the length, configuration, and support of the bladder neck and urethra affording continence. It allows an assessment of the presence of outside pressure on the bladder from other structures, i.e. a large fibroid or ovarian cyst pushing on the bladder and thereby compromising capacity, and the ballooning of the bladder from the collapse of the front vaginal wall support into a cysotocoele. The examination is uncomfortable, but tolerable, and can be completed in only a few minutes. Recent data indicate cystourethroscopy is not a necessary part of the evaluation of the patient with stress incontinence solely to assess the bladder outlet in stress incontinence. It is often used, as previously mentioned, in the evaluation particularly if there are other concerns, for example, hematuria

These tests will provide the data base upon which the choice of treatment, pharmacologic or surgical, is made.

TREATMENT

Treatment regimens fall into three categories: behavior modification, medication, and surgery. These also allow a progressive treatment based upon the severity of the condition and the particular type of bladder and support which the patient possesses (Recall Sharon and Marcella.). Ultimately, the treatment decision, especially if surgery is contemplated, depends upon how socially limiting the problem is to the woman. If her urinary habits limit or severely affect the way she goes about her day, i.e. she has stopped taking her afternoon walk because of the fear of wetness, certainly treatment, even involving surgery, would be indicated. This parallels the decision making process made by men with prostate gland enlargement.

Behavior modification involves attentiveness to timely bladder emptying and elimination of bladder irritants, i.e. caffeine, nicotine (cigarettes), excessive spicy foods and chocolate. A technique of timed, double-voiding has been previously described to emptying the bladder as well as possible before engaging in activities during which leakage is more likely to occur. Kegel exercises may assist in milder cases.

Pharmacologic treatment (medications) are generally employed in three ways. First is to assist the neck of the bladder to tighten maximally. As mentioned previously, these medications are the common cold preparations, i.e. Actifed® or Sudafed®, (alpha adrenergics) and can be used on an as needed basis when leakage is most likely to occur. Taken too frequently or regularly for a prolonged basis, they are prone to elevate the blood pressure and/or to lose their effectiveness. These preparations should be employed with the behavior modification techniques mentioned above.

Second, if the bladder has elevated pressure or instability (involuntary contractions) both noted as urgency to urinate by the patient, i.e. from radiation irritation or chronic irritation from recurring infections, medications which relax the bladder may yield dryness. These medications must be used with caution in patients with glaucoma and also can cause a troublesome dryness of mouth, sun sensitivity, and constipation.

Third, approximately 10% of women will have incontinence after menopause, increasing with age. Estrogen therapy softens the urethra, improving its closure properties, and increases certain receptors in the woven muscle at the bladder neck and first portion of the urethra making the urethra more susceptible to alpha adrenergics (See above). Up to two-thirds report reduced urge incontinence, but there is little evidence to support the use of estrogens alone to improve stress incontinence. Precautions for endometrial cancer include cyclic administration (like birth control pill cycling) and use of progesterone as well. There is slightly increased risk of gall bladder disease and possibly high blood pressure.

The goals of any surgical treatment for stress urinary incontinence in females are:

> 1.) To reconstitute the normal angle (position and support) between the urethra and the bladder and the fixation between the urethra and pelvic floor, thereby
> 2.) Lengthening the urethra, and
> 3.) In accomplishing (2.), tightening the urethra;

Goals 2 and 3 are applications of simple fluid fluid laws of physics which state that resistance to flow is increased and less flow is likely to occur, in a longer tube than a shorter one. Additionally, as a diameter of a tube is halved, the resistance to flow is not just doubled, it is increased by a factor to its fourth power or 16 fold! Remember the female urethra as a Chinese finger trap. As we pull upon it surgically to lengthen it, we tighten it as well, thus accomplishing our second two goals.

Angles are important in anatomy. The angle, or position and support, between the bladder and urethra is such that as forces are generated in the abdomen, they are directed at the neck of the bladder in such way that it actually tightens or coapts the neck to close it tighter, much like a baffle valve. With stress incontinence this angulation is lost because the urethra is allowed to migrate. The pressure generated in the abdomen as a result of lifting or laughing pushes the mobile urethra down and makes it shorter and wider and thus incompetent to maintain dryness, much in the manner by which we remove our fingers from the Chinese finger trap. We push the fingers together to shorten the woven tube and to widen it. Surgical correction fixes the urethra to maintain its angulation and to prevent its mobility and foreshortening.

However, anatomic support alone may not be sufficient to achieve continence, particularly if the intrinsic urethral resistance is lost. The intrinsic urethral resistance is the contribution to dryness which comes from the simple coaptation (closure) and support of the spongy urethral tissue, particularly at the most proximal urethra adjoining the bladder neck.

There are many surgical procedures to accomplish the goals within both the urologic and gynecologic armamentarium. The classic procedure performed, through an abdominal incision, places stitches into the tough tissue around the neck of the bladder and tacks this tissue to the underside of the pubic bone (See Figure 10-2). This repair, named the Marshall-Marchetti-Krantz Procedure or MMK for short, was the standard repair performed for many years and is still widely used particularly if other procedures are planned through the abdominal incision, i.e. removal of the womb (hysterectomy).

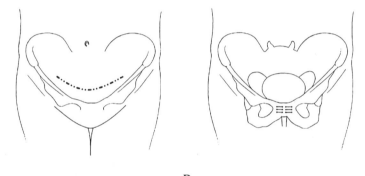

A.   B.

Figure 10-2: The Marshall-Marchetti-Krantz (MMK) Procedure.

Vaginal repairs are frequently performed to repair associated anatomic problems as well, i.e. repair of a cysotocoele and/or rectocoele (protrusions of the front and/or back wall of the vagina in which is/are the bladder and/or rectum). Urologists also perform a vaginal support, as a group called endoscopic urethral suspension procedures (See Figure 10-3). Several have been described (for example, the Stamey procedure, the Raz procedure, and the Gittes procedure) but in each, through small vaginal incision(s), the tissues to each side of the neck of the bladder are used to be "suspended" by sutures (stitches) to the muscle layers of the abdominal wall. This is performed through a small incision made slightly above the pubic bone below the hair line, thus rendering a much more cosmetically acceptable

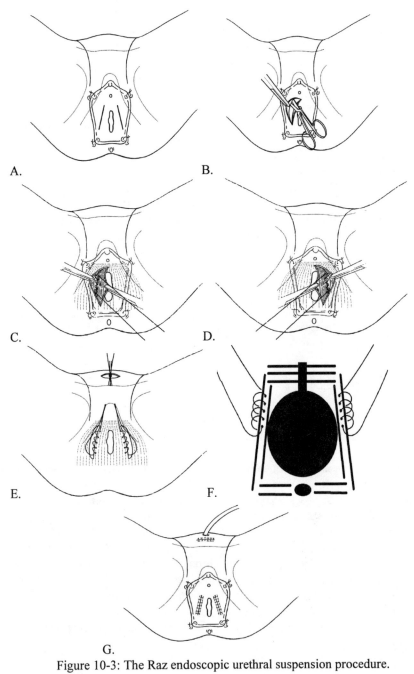

A.

B.

C.

D.

E.

F.

G.

Figure 10-3: The Raz endoscopic urethral suspension procedure.

surgery.   Long needles are placed through the abdominal incision and directed behind the pubic bone through the vaginal incision. The sutures are then drawn up through the abdominal incision and tied in place, suspending the neck of the bladder by the "tummy" muscles. Think of the reins of a horse, offering some resistance all the time, but taut as the muscles tighten with any lifting, straining, or lifting.

As an aside, a woman with only a vaginal repair of a cystocoele planned may occasionally manifest with stress incontinence following her surgery when she resumes normal activities. The reason for this is that the vaginal protrusion served as a "pop-off" valve which, previous to the repair, alleviated the pressure on the bladder and prevented leakage. Now, without that "pop-off", she leaks to varying degrees. Therefore, in order to prevent this frustration and need for additional surgery, attentiveness to a urologic evaluation prior and good bladder neck support at the time of surgery is performed, frequently involving a joint gynecologic/urologic repair.

Length of disability or limitation may vary, but within a few weeks relatively normal activities with the exception of no lifting or straining, and within six weeks or so incremental increases of activities can be resumed. By 10 to 12 weeks after the procedure, full activities can be resumed.

Success rates of better than 90% at two years after the procedure are achieved. The "proof in the pudding" for a surgical repair is the 5 year period. Currently, endoscopic supports seem to yield superior results, with better than 80% maintaining dryness at 5 years, depending upon the degree of incontinence before surgery.

There are three additional surgical approaches for stress available. First, minimally invasive and effective for carefully selected patients is the injection in and around the bladder neck through the cystoscope of collagen (a normal body protein) or of fat (harvested by suction from our fatty tissues). Important to understand is the need for multiple and repeat injections. Second, a "sling" procedure is one in which a band of the patient's own tissue, usually the tough tissue called fascia over the abdominal muscles, is constructed as a sling or wrap around the bladder neck to assist dryness. Thirdly, in severe cases of total lack of support, the artificial sphincter can be placed (See Figure 9-4, in Bladder Basics).

SUMMARY

Dryness is achievable for most patients through a variety of treatments including behavior modification, medication, and surgery. As with most conditions, equal attentiveness to detail by both the patient and the physician is key to a successful outcome. For the patient, eliminating cigarette smoking, for instance, could eliminate chronic cough and make a successful outcome more likely to be sustained. For the gynecologist or urologist, assuring a clear understanding of the patient's bladder function is critical. Together as a team, resuming of normal activities without concern for wetness is achievable.

CHAPTER 11

URETHRAL STENOSIS

Bladder irritability, particularly in women after menopause.

A very common condition affecting post-menopausal women is the syndrome of urethral stenosis and chronic cystitis. Men should read this chapter as well, for two reasons. First, many of the principles involved parallel those associated with prostate problems in men. Secondly, men are frequently impatient and fail to acknowledge that their spouse's or friend's "weak bladder" is a very real medical condition. The common complaints experienced by these women are urgency, occasional urge incontinence, frequency, and nocturia. Urgency is the sudden unannounced feeling of an immediate need to urinate, many times resulting in the inability to get to a bathroom in time yielding wetting or urge incontinence. Frequency is obviously urinating more frequently than one is accustomed. Nocturia is the need to urinate during sleeping hours and is frequently associated with bedwetting or nocturnal enuresis.

A stenosis is a narrowing or tightening. The urethra is the tube connecting the bladder to the outside of the body. As a result of menopause--whether it be natural, surgical (as a result of removal of the ovaries), or chemical--the female genitalia, which depend upon balanced hormonal status, begin to atrophy and tighten down. The most dramatic changes occur in the introitus (vaginal opening) and vaginal walls themselves. Frequently, the urethra, which lies in the anterior or top vaginal wall, is entrapped in this process and is compressed or squeezed. In severe cases, the urethra itself becomes fibrosed or scarred. The result of this process is a tighter tube through which the urine must be pushed to empty the bladder. This process is a very gradual one, taking many years to develop so the bladder has a very gradual response to the need to generate more pressure to empty itself.

Remember from our discussion of the bladder anatomy and function, it is literally a hollow muscle with a reserve to work extra hard when necessary. Think of the bladder as Arnold Schwartzenegger's arms. As a result of the years of hard work, his arms are sculptures of every muscle fiber grouped into bundles. Each muscle is readily apparent. Also, Arnold is unable to relax his arms totally down to his side because of their tautness. So it is with the

91

bladder which has been subjected to a narrowing urethra over years. It too has worked hard, and it too has thickened its muscles and become more taut. As a result , the bladder is unable to stretch as it did when it was soft and compliant, then cannot hold as much urine as it did many years before. The patient goes to the bathroom more frequently because the capacity is reduced, yielding daytime frequency and nighttime voiding.

Contributing as well to the frequency and nocturia is the fact that even though the bladder may feel empty, it really has a significant amount of residual urine(that left at the completion of voiding). This results because the muscles of the bladder can push only so much and so long before giving up. What many women experience is dribbling throughout or near completion of voiding as the bladder tires.If they wait several seconds to a few minutes, they are able to void an additional amount of urine because that bladder has rested and is able to be worked again.

Now look what has happened! We have crimped the ability of the bladder at the high end by not being able to hold as much, and that which are able to hold we don't empty completely. The functional volume, or that volume through which we work on a daily basis, is severely compromised and these women literally are tethered to the toilet.

There is an additional factor which contributes to this problem. The normal resting pressure in the bladder is approximately 15 centimeters of water. Don't worry about the units, just remember the number 15. The healthy young woman with no bladder problems urinates with an average pressure of somewhere around 30. As a result of the bladder muscles becoming taut from chronic overworking in urethral stenosis, the resting pressure in many of these women's bladders may be 40, 50, even 60 centimeters of water. In other words, these women at rest have significantly more pressure in their bladder than the healthy young woman during urination. It's no wonder they experience almost a continual sensation to urinate, or an urge to race to the bathroom when they hear water running.

Recall from our discussion in Chapter 9 of the interaction between the bladder and the brain, the brain is constantly telling the bladder to relax. When urination does occur, it is because the brain"looks the other way" and "allows" urination to occur, more than telling it to do so. The symptoms of urgency, frequency, urge incontinence, and nocturia in elderly women are likely from changes in the central nervous system's inhibitory influences, as well.

As a result of the residual urine left in the bladder on a chronic basis, the women with urethral stenosis are prone to recurrent, or repeat, urinary tract infections. Any time we don't readily purge a body fluid, there is risk for infection, i.e. pneumonia is likely to occur when a portion of the lung fails to clear its secretions readily. Bladder infections irritate the bladder sending false messages to the brain, messages which are interpreted as the need to void. This then worsens already bothersome symptoms.

With all this bad news, what can we do to help?

If we assume the cause to be one of a blockage or narrowing of the tube which conducts the urine from the bladder to its exit, the most direct treatment would address this blockage.

Estrogen therapy can counteract vaginal atrophy. It can also soften the urethra and thereby improve its closure properties by improving the urethra's blood supply and reversing the decline in healthy protein called collagen. Also, estrogen therapy makes the urethra more sensitive to alpha adrenergic medications or common cold preparations, like Sudafed® and Actifed®, if incontinence is a problem. Estrogens do reduce urge incontinence in up to two-thirds of patients, but they do not improve stress urinary incontinence. One must consider the risks of long-term therapy of estrogens including endometrial cancer (in women with a uterus), gallbladder disease, blood-clotting disease, and elevated blood pressure.

Many of these women will benefit from an outpatient or office procedure wherein the urethra is dilated or stretched by the sequential passage of probes (called "sounds") through the urethra into the bladder. Under a local anesthetic, like your dentist uses but in a gel form, the tube is numbed. The sounds are inserted one at a time in increasing size until a suitable dilation of the tube has occurred. Most urologists today discourage the once-popular practice of frequent dilation. With the development of several medications which can complement dilation, we are now able to avoid the pitfalls inherent in repeated instrumentation. With frequent dilation a vicious cycle is induced: dilation leads to inflammation which leads to scarification (scar development) which results in even worse stenosis requiring repeat dilation. Most urologists who perform dilation favor a rare but occasional dilation to interrupt the necessity of high pressure voiding. Over time (anywhere usually from 6 to 12 weeks) after the dilation, the bladder "learns" that it doesn't have to work so hard to empty its contents. As a result of lower pressures during voiding (micturition), the bladder also "learns" to rest at lower pressures. With lower pressures at rest the constant urge to void is dramatically improved. With lowered resting pressures, these women are not as likely to be awakened at night with the sudden urge to urinate. Their sleep is also less likely to be interrupted because their bladders can now relax and hold more, and that which they are able to hold is more completely expelled because they are no longer voiding against a tight resistance. Their "functional volume" has been increased. Finally, as a result of more complete emptying they are less likely to develop urinary tract infections because there is less retained urine to serve as a nice rich culture medium should the bladder become contaminated--as female bladders particularly are more common to have occur.

If life were only this simple!

In reality this problem in women and prostatitis in men comprise what I call the "low back pain" of urology. By that I mean that these problems serve as a nemesis for the patient and the physician. The patients become easily frustrated because of the lengthy symptoms, because of the tendency for the problem to recur once addressed, and many times because of the frustration of the physician who is in the business of attempting to help someone but seemingly finds his success short-lived or even completely thwarted

Fortunately, as I alluded to above, many new medications have improved our ability to treat this condition. Many urologists will add bladder relaxants to treat these patients if suitable results are not obtained by dilation or estrogen therapy alone. Approximately two thirds do see improvement after dilation. To those who are not improved at all (whose bladder will remain taut even in the face of reduced pressure necessary to void) or who have not obtained a suitable degree of improvement, the use of a bladder relaxant may make the situation more bearable and prevent their urinary habits from continuing to be a social hindrance. In this setting it is particularly important to "success"! The woman cannot logically expect her bladder to behave as it did when she was 25. But if we can keep the urgency as "background noise" or a minor aggravation rather than "right up front" and distracting, if we can keep the number of trips to the restroom socially acceptable, albeit more frequently than she would really like, then that will have to be called "success". I have many women who function quite nicely taking their bladder relaxant only when they are to be out and about, whether at work, running errands, or socially. When they are at home then they don't take their medication and "live with" more frequent trips to the bathroom.

Many women who are bothered only with being awakened several times per night but experience little daytime inconvenience do quite well by taking their bladder relaxant at bedtime only.

Again defining what is to called "success" is important. The woman who is "beckoned" from her sleep 6 to 8 times per night must call getting up twice "success".

A final word of clarification is in order. The dilation procedure which we've spoken of here is of the urethra and not of the bladder (as performed in diseases of the bladder primarily which compromise its ability to serve as suitable reservoir). And while, indeed, the dilation procedure is simple and performed in the office setting, a complete urologic evaluation is in order for the patient first presenting to the urologist's office. While it is true that the majority of women with this symptom complex will have "only" urethral stenosis, other much more devastating diseases including cancer of the bladder may also be present. Therefore, most urologists will accompany the dilation with a cystoscopy, or look in the bladder, to rule-out these other more occult problems. If from the history there appears to be a concern regarding a possible neurologic (nerve) problem or a more complex incontinence situation involving both urge and stress incontinence components, then a full complement of bladder tone testing, called urodynamics, may be ordered. Obviously then the evaluation and treatment is tailored to the patient based upon the initial history and physical exam. Once established, these steps do not need to be repeated unless there are changes in the history which would dictate otherwise, such as newly developed signs of blood in the urine or numerous urinary tract infections.

CHAPTER 12

INTERSTITIAL CYSTITIS

Bladder irritability, particularly in younger women.

Classically described as "angry patients with angry bladders", these are among the most frustrated patients in a urologic practice. Symptoms are generally marked urinary frequency during both day and night and pain (in the area just above the pubic bone at the lower portion of our abdomen)-- especially upon bladder filling and at the completion of voiding as the pressure in the bladder has been sustained to empty. Frequently the symptoms reach their final stage rapidly and may be sustained for years. While several causes have been proposed, interstitial cysitis may be related to an immune-type reaction following an infection, specifically to a bacteria called the Streptococcus, although the urine remains sterile on multiple cultures performed in the course of evaluation and treatment. There might be defects in the lining of the bladder or even family inheritance patterns have been suggested.

The clinical condition frequently occurs in Type A individuals (the more high-strung or "driven" individuals), although many investigators feel the condition itself is so consuming that it can result in personality upsets for the patients rendering them "high strung". Females outnumber males approximately 10 to 1, and it frequently occurs in women who have had previous pelvic surgery. This psychologically very stressful condition frequently occurs in individuals who are otherwise healthy and active but who can truly become "bladder invalids" from pain, urgency (sudden, severe need to urinate), and frequency.

While the diagnosis is suspected from the patient's history, an evaluation will often include a cystoscopy, or look in the bladder, possibly with bladder biopsies performed with special instrumentation through the cystoscope. Frequently, as this procedure is performed under anesthesia, an initial treatment option of those discussed below will be included in that procedure. Biopsies are considered to assure the accuracy of the diagnosis and to rule-out the remote possibility of a bladder cancer, particularly in most males and female patients older than 50 wherein that diagnosis becomes more likely (See Chapter 14, Bladder Cancer and Blood in the Urine). In other words, males at any age with symptoms of prolonged bladder irritation are 10 times more likely to have bladder cancer than females. Females, particularly if under age 45 to 50, are more likely to have interstitial cystitis with similar symptoms. After age 50 in females, the diagnosis of bladder cancer becomes more likely than intestitial cystitis; but females have less bladder cancer overall than males. Interestingly, the incidence of bladder cancer in females has continued to approach that of males over the last several decades. Nonetheless, viewing the bladder directly and consideration of biopsy will eliminate an error in diagnosis.

Treatment includes:

1.) systemic treatment (medications taken orally or by injection which are distributed throughout the body) as one would treat any inflammatory condition, i.e. steroids, antihistamines, and non-steroidal antiinflammatories;

2.) local treatment to the bladder, i.e. distention or stretching of the bladder under anesthesia, instillation into the bladder of various chemicals including DMSO, steroids, and heparin; infiltration by injection of steroids into the bladder wall;

3.) surgery or injection therapy to denervate the bladder, that is, to strip or inactivate the nerves which mediate painful sensations from the bladder;

4.) bladder substitution or urinary diversion in which the bladder is removed and either a new bladder is constructed by using portions of the patient's intestine or the urine is directed into an appliance worn on the belly wall by use of a piece of patient's intestine.

It stands to reason that if there are this many treatment options available for a disease, any disease, we really don't understand its cause. If we did, we would develop and direct the "magic bullet" to treat it. While in fact the clinical complaints of the patient are fairly characteristic, the appearance of the bladder when viewed through the cystoscope is fairly characteristic, and the biopsies of the bladder are fairly characteristic when looked at under the microscope, we do not know its cause. Therefore, the success of any treatment is limited. Frequently, despite whatever treatment(s) is(are) selected, only time will allow the resolution of this process. However, only 10% can be expected to spontaneously (without treatment) resolve their disease.The goal of therapy, especially in the young patient, with early disease, is to apply the least invasive treatment of afford reasonable symptomatic relief. The recurrent and chronic nature of this disease results in the need for continuous or intermittent treatment. In the meantime, these patients require tremendous reassurance and support because this disease truly is as painful and frustrating as any chronic pain condition, i.e. back problems or hip problems.

For more information write or call: The Interstitial Cystitis Association, P.O. Box 1553, Madison Square Station, New York, NY, 10159; (212) 979-6057.

CHAPTER 13

BEDWETTING

Causes and treatments of bedwetting.

No topic serves as a more volatile source of problems in an otherwise tranquil home than bedwetting (nocturnal enuresis). Besides the tremendous inconvenience it causes with the continual change of bedding or the need to wake the sleeping child to attempt to urinate, it is frequently mistaken as manipulative behavior, possibly making an already tense home setting worse.

The best way to defuse this potentially explosive situation is to understand its causes and then to avoid those things which might make it more likely to occur. At age 5 years, approximately 15% of children are enuretic, a majority of whom have nocturnal enuresis. The bottom line is that no matter what is done, the problem resolves at a rate of approximately 15% per year even if no treatment is rendered. This gives promise that the problem will resolve fairly easily in majority of cases; however, most urologists have at least a few adult patients, otherwise healthy and active, who suffer this malady.

Recall from our discussion of the interaction between the bladder and the central nervous system (See Bladder Basics, Chapter 9), the brain serves as a continuous deterrent to the bladder's expelling its contents. In other words, urination occurs as the brain releases its control and allows the bladder to function automatically. During times of filling, the brain must continually tell the bladder, "No! No! Not yet!" until the appropriate, socially acceptable time at which point the brain "looks the other way" and the bladder seizes the opportunity for spontaneous urination to occur. During certain phases of sleep, the brain's control is lax or lost, and wetting occurs with bedwetters. This is more likely to occur if the bladder is full--and therefore occurs most frequently several hours after bedtime. We cannot address the brain's developing ability to control the bladder in the treatment of bedwetting. We can, however, alter several other factors which will lessen the bladder's likelihood of functioning automatically.

The easiest treatments are in the form of simple behavior modification techniques. These children should be made to understand that this is their problem--that it is not just happening to them, and therefore they are the key participants to any reasonable solutions. They are the ones sleeping in the wet bed and clothing, and they are the ones subject to cruel jokes from their peers should the problem not be corrected before they begin to spend nights at friends' homes or travel. This can be communicated to the child in a caring, concerned way and does not have to be threatening. In making this very clear at the outset, however, these children understand very clearly that they must be very active in any successful treatment. Relying upon parents, an occasional visit to the physician's office, or a pill is not going to correct the problem. In my practice I make certain the child hears this from me. Many are in an age where they will be able to "cheat" because they are not under 100% observation--nor should they need to be. The keeping of a voiding diary or log of nights wet/dry also facilitates better motivation for the child and provides visual feedback for the success or failure of other behavior modifications described below. It also allows a tangible measurement for the parents to establish goals which are mutually agreed upon for reward, i.e. a trip to the local toy store for a small treat for seven consecutive nights of dryness.

Bedwetters should first limit their fluids after dinner. There is an agreement of sorts between the parents and the child as to what the amount should be and that's it for the evening. Preferably, limited fluids are ingested within 2 hours (and certainly very strictly limited within 1 hour) of bedtime. This obviously is an effort to relatively dehydrate the child through the sleeping hours so that the bladder is filled more slowly.

In addition, the child is asked to "double-void" before bedtime. This is not some strange way of urinating in two streams at once. Double-voiding simply is a technique used in an attempt to assure that the bladder is as empty as it can be. The technique is to void approximately 20 to 30 minutes prior to bedtime and then to return for a second attempt right at bedtime. This technique is used to start the night with a "dry" bladder, and in doing so to prevent filling to the point where the bladder wants to empty automatically until a time when the brain is no longer in its deepest stages of sleep. As the bedwetter emerges from these deep stages of sleep, the brain is able to once again exert its control over the bladder.

Another technique to accomplish this delay in filling is to awaken the child at the parent's bedtime which is usually at least a few hours later. Alarms can be used to awaken the child as wetting is initiated. Both of these can be disruptive to the household because the child may be frequently irritable if not combative. Reiterating the concept of the child as a participant in the treatment, they the need to get themselves out of bed and to the restroom should they awaken from sleep for any reason. All of the above techniques are useful because on a percentage basis the most likely time for a child to wet is between 3 A.M. and 6 A.M. If we can get them through this time interval with some capacity reserve, they are likely to be awakened themselves to urinate through their own internal alarm.

There are some additional behavior modification techniques which are important as well. I ask the parents and children to entirely eliminate caffeine from the bedwetter's diet. With soft drinks now in all combinations of sugar-free and caffeine-free, this is less of a sacrifice than it used to be. Nonetheless, the child who is of an age that he or she is independent may cheat on this. I stress that even daytime caffeine should be eliminated. Also surprising is the number of young children who drink coffee and tea. Most tea products have a higher caffeine content than coffee. With both (and don't forget iced tea), caffeine-free products are also available.

Chocolate should also be placed "on waivers" with bedwetters. Now you're only a kid once, and I rank right up there as with some of the all-time "chocoholics", but certainly excesses should be eliminated. I've yet to read any scientific data on this, but my teaching was and my clinical experience has been by the elimination of excessive chocolate consumption bedwetting may be improved most probably again by elimination of the additional caffeine.

Assuming a child with an otherwise normal medical history, normal physical exam, and normal urinalysis (urine check), behavior modification techniques are given 6 to 8 weeks. This draws the child into the process and makes them a participant . A majority of patients will note improvement, if not complete resolution of the problem, by that time. If no significant progress has been made at that point and the child and parents are content that no improvement in behavior is needed, then medications which assist in buying additional bladder capacity are used.

The anticholinergics or bladder relaxants are a group of medications which best accomplish this increase in bladder capacity to get the bedwetter through their most vulnerable time (a bladder filled to near capacity during a time of deep sleep). Oxybutynin (Ditropan®) and hyoscamine (Levsin® or Anaspaz®) are two members of this group which may be used with success. The side-effects of these medications include a dryness of mouth (these medications are also sometimes used to dry secretions before general anesthesia), but this is not too bothersome because the child is sleeping when the medication level is highest. Fair children will also be more sensitive to the sun. Success rates of 60 to 80% are achievable.

Imipramine (Tofranil®) has also been widely used in this setting. It acts as a direct bladder relaxant but it also works in the central nervous system in a not completely understood way. The main side-effect of this medication is that the children do complain of feeling tired or sluggish, of dryness of mouth and sun sensitivity, and some parents note changes in the child's personality while the medication is used.

As an aside, you may have heard of Tofranil® being used for depression, and indeed this whole group, called the tricyclic antidepressants, are used in the treatment of schizophrenia and depression. This explains why many patients with these psychiatric problems may also have urinary problems, mainly incontinence. Worsening their overall general inattentiveness to their normal bowel and bladder bodily functions is a treatment which tends to weaken the bladder's ability to empty itself when full and increases their thirst as a side-effect thereby increasing their urine output. What results is "overflow" incontinence, wherein the bladder is stretched beyond its ability to hold any more and beyond its capability to contract and expel its contents. Therefore it just leaks all the time. A parallel condition can occur with bowel habits.

We do not advocate use of Tofranil® for bedwetting because of its side-effects despite its nearly 70% success rate. If behavior modification and first line medications don't succeed, then DDAVP® (a type of vasopressin or water conserving compound) may be employed. This medication works on the principle that, during times of dehydration, our bodies will preserve fluids in our systems by "instructing" the kidneys to make the urine very concentrated. This is accomplished through a very complicated series of steps by specialized hormones (chemicals produced and released into our bloodstream which act at a distant site to turn on a specific function, i.e. control of the kidneys). DDAVP® signals the kidneys to re-absorb a large percentage of the water back into the bloodstream. The end result is that the volume of urine made is less, and the system has restored a large percentage of the volume which otherwise would have been lost. DDAVP® is the synthetic, or manufactured, mediator of this process. Its success in the treatment of bedwetting then is to lessen the amount of urine being presented to the bladder during sleep in an attempt to delay bladder filling through the period of sleep when the "internal alarm" is least likely to arouse the child.

DDAVP® is an excellent tool to have for use, but many feel that, although all studies indicate it is safe, it should be used when other less physiologically harsh methods have failed. It is expensive and adverse reactions, while limited, do include nasal congestion, flushing, headaches, and abdominal cramps. We have used it very successfully in the older child or adult with wetting. It is a nasal spray, and therefore can be problematic with compliance with the younger child.

Bedwetting will be solved for an overwhelming percentage of patients, even if only through that achieved by the passage of time. However, one must always be watchful of other associated signs or symptoms which may point to an underlying problem which results in bedwetting as a symptom, i.e. daytime accidents suggesting a potential neurologic (nerve) problem or infection. Associated bowel problems may indicate similarly neurologic problem. Bowel and bladder problems are common ways in which childhood psychiatric problems manifest themselves. And, even if under successful management, any child seen at the doctor's office being treated for enuresis should have a urinalysis (urine check) to make certain there is no infection or blood under the microscope, which again would suggest that the bedwetting was a symptom of another problem.

Once successful, depending upon the age of the child, after several months the treatment may be gradually eliminated. Through this time, and in many cases into adulthood, the child will continue to employ those behavior modification techniques which were used as the foundation of the treatment. For at least a few years the child may require medication to take, if he or she wishes, for overnight stays, outings, or on trips--any situation which presents a change of their normal routine and which would be embarrassing for the bedwetter to have a setback.

Remember parents of bedwetters: if one parent was a wetter, the likelihood of a child wetting is 50%. If both parents were wetters, the likelihood is 70%. When your child, the bedwetter, is toiling with your grandchild over bedwetting, remind her or him of this "inheritance" and the positive manner with which you approached this problem!

For more information write or call: The National Enuresis Society, P.O. Box 6351, Parsippany, N.J., 07054; (800) NES-8080.

CHAPTER 14

BLOOD IN THE URINE AND BLADDER CANCER

Conditions causing blood in the urine; and, cancer of the bladder.

It's time to think of a urologist's (or any physician's) job in almost a philosophical sense. Our job is first as a physician, second as a surgeon, and third as a surgical specialist. In listening to a patient's complaints or reviewing labwork or xrays, we think of the likely diagnoses; that is, those diagnoses which are most likely to yield those complaints or results in testing. What separates the average from the astute clinician is in not assuming that the likely diagnosis is accounting for the results, but rather in thinking of those diagnoses which, while not as likely, if missed could yield a very bad outcome for the patient. These diagnoses are ruled out by further testing which is hopefully minimally invasive and cost effective. One good example is President Reagan's hemorrhoids! If his physicians had assumed that the bleeding he was experiencing was attributable to his hemorrhoids, his colon cancer upstream would have been missed and possibly no cure could have been rendered with a delayed diagnosis. His evaluation included the additional testing by colonoscopy (an outpatient, local anesthetic look in the large bowel), and the tumor was discovered early.

GENERAL PRINCIPLES

And so it is with blood in the urine (hematuria, hema=blood,+ uria=urine)-- even if only under the microscope. All blood in the urine requires concern and possibly full urologic evaluation including an IVP (intravenous pyelogram or xray of the kidneys) if the kidney function is adequate and a cystoscopy (look in the bladder with a scope of either rigid or flexible type). If the blood is assumed to be accountable because of an infection of the bladder or of the prostate gland or a kidney stone for instance (See Chapter 24, Infection of the Urinary Tract and Chapter 17, Kidney Stones), then subsequent checks of the urine once that condition has cleared or has been treated should show no further blood. Persistence of the blood, even if only under the microscope (microscopic hematuria) is reason to suggest an evaluation.

Visible blood generally denotes a more active, vigorous process. Blood initially in the urinary stream which clears as urination continues suggests a lower source, i.e. of the urethra (tube connecting the bladder to the outside) or prostate gland. The blood is purged or washed away with urination. Blood throughout urination suggests bladder or kidney sources. Long, slender clots suggests blood which has clotted in the ureter (tube connecting the kidney to the bladder). This discussion really is academic, however, as any bleeding would warrant a full evaluation, stem to stern.

Blood under the microscope requires more attentiveness to its collection in order to eliminate the possibility of a false positive urinalysis. Translation: the urine may show some microscopic hematuria if the patient has been very physically active, i.e. jogging, within 24 hours of its submission. Therefore, anything strenuous or jarring activities and intercourse should be avoided to eliminate any contribution from those activities which may be minimally traumatizing to the kidneys, bladder or urethra yet significant enough to have some blood cells shed into the urine from a break in the integrity of their lining. If, on multiple checks performed over several weeks, it has failed to clear, evaluation is in order.

With microscopic hematuria, one completed evaluation negative for malignancy (cancer) or other identifiable causes for blood does not free the patient from future concern. The hypothesis has to be proposed: what if something is present, like a very early cancer, which is neither detectable by xray nor by cystoscopy? If true, it would "fester" into a detectable lesion which could be seen either by xray or by a look in the bladder within a year or so. Therefore, following a negative IVP and cystoscopy, most urologists would suggest continued checks of the urine by urinalysis. If the checks continue to show blood, even under the microscope only, then a repeat evaluation would be warranted in 6 to 12 months. Two evaluations spaced roughly one year apart, both negative, frees the patient as close to 100% certainty as we can be that cancer is accounting for the blood. Should, however, the patient pass visible blood at any time, an evaluation is once again warranted. In my own practice, I have a patient who was negative at an evaluation performed in 1988 for microscopic hematuria. By 1990, upon presenting to me after moving to our area and without any interim follow-up per the patient's decision, she presented with visible blood in her urine and was discovered to have a sizeable kidney cancer. She ultimately has done well, but not without significantly compromising that outcome because of her reluctance to seek follow-up until the condition was dire.

One diagnosis outside of the urinary tract warranting discussion is tuberculosis. Particularly if the patient has been or has been around incarcerated individuals, institutionalized individuals, or other patients of T.B., tuberculosis should be entertained as a diagnosis. The urinary tract is the number one system outside of the lungs to become infected with the tuberculin organism. T.B. incidence is on the upswing, and its presence also indicates the need for AIDS testing (See Chapter 28, AIDS). The evaluation is the PPD (skin test) and a chest xray.

Blood in the urine associated with other symptoms may suggest a diagnosis. For instance, if a patient experiences a sudden onset of urgency, frequency, and fever, an infection is suggested possibly of the bladder, kidneys, or prostate (in males). If the patient is experiencing severe loin or flank pain, possibly a kidney stone is in passage. If the patient has experienced several weeks of loss of appetite and/or weight, possibly a cancer of the bladder or kidney is present. Nonetheless, despite what differential diagnoses may be suggested by the nature of the bleeding or associated symptoms, the work-up is the same for each and includes the IVP and a cystoscopy. Subsequently, additional tests may be required, i.e. a CT Scan of the kidneys, based upon a suggestion of a problem on the initial studies.

For hematuria, the IVP and the cystoscopy remain the "gold standard" first tests. Again, the only exceptions to performing an IVP would be concern about:

      1.) the patient's kidney function being able to handle the contrast (xray "dye"),
      2.) if the patient is severely dehydrated,
      3.) if the the patient has a contrast allergy, or
      4.) in special situations, for instance where the protein in the urine is high, where the test could not be safely administered.

Cystoscopic instruments are both rigid and flexible, each with advantages and disadvantages. Both can be employed with a minimal amount of discomfort and using only a local anesthetic, if only a "look-see" is to be performed. For more extensive procedures, i.e. biopsies or stone manipulations, then regional or general anesthetics may be required.

The different diagnoses are discussed in their respective chapters including prostate causes in Chapters 7, 8, and 25; bladder causes in Chapters 9, 11, 12,

14,and 24, kidney causes in Chapters 16 and 17; and venereal (sexually transmitted disease) causes in Chapter 26.

BLADDER CANCER

Bladder cancer is a skin cancer--of the special skin lining (called transitional cell epithelium) of the bladder. With growth, it may bleed, cause irritation in the bladder mimicking the urge to urinate, or serve as a sticky location for bacteria to adhere, multiply, and cause further irritation by infection. Any cell layer of our body which has a rapid turnover rate (that is, the cells form, grow, and die fairly rapidly) are more prone to an error in the genetic message occurring and a cancer resulting. Other examples are the lining of the lungs and the lining of the large bowel (colon). There are certain factors which are linked as causative: certain dyes (Note hairdressers or workers in the dye industry!), certain chemicals particularly in the rubber industry, analgesic abuse (particularly phenacetin), and SMOKING. Smokers have a 40 to 200 times the general population incidence of bladder cancer, and the risk goes even higher if that risk is in addition to others, i.e. a smoking hairdresser. Men are more likely (approximately 3:1), yet as more women smoke, this gap is closing. The incidence is seemingly increasing, yet it is unclear whether this is a true increase in the disease or having more patients alerted to the signs and symptoms and therefore seeking evaluation.

Approximately 50,000 new cases are diagnosed each year. About 10,000 die from their disease each year. In 1993, bladder cancer will account for nearly 10% of new cancer diagnoses in males (5% for females), and for the same year the disease will have accounted for 3 to 5% of cancer deaths among adults. Our mortality figures do reflect an improvement in survival over the last several years.

The best way to think of bladder cancer is as "the tumor of two-thirds". Approximately two-thirds will recur (have another tumor); of those, two-thirds will survive their disease (conversely, one-third will die from their disease). Two-thirds will successfully respond to "first line" chemical treatments placed in the bladder (intravesicle chemotherapy); of those who fail, two thirds will respond to a second line of chemical treatments. Two-thirds will recur with a lesion of equal or less anger under the microscope, but one-third will recur with a more aggressive tumor. In summary, taking care of bladder cancer is like pulling weeds from your garden. You just have to keep pulling them until you get ahead to prevent their coming back; it's easier to pull them when they're few and small, and you occasionally have to use chemical treatments to prevent them from growing back.

Sizeable tumors of the bladder may be seen on the IVP however, the IVP alone is not sufficient to evaluate the bladder. Because of its shape, the bladder filled with contrast from the IVP may obscure a tumor in the bladder as it is surrounded on all sides by contrast. Even with a normal IVP, a look in the bladder with the cystoscope is necessary. This is usually performed with a local anesthetic, i.e. Xylocaine® jelly is placed down the urethra. If there is strong suspicion of a tumor on xray, however, the urologist may suggest an anesthetic, either regional (spinal) or general, which would allow the lesion to be biopsied and or removed (resected) through the cystoscope during the initial instrumentation.

Three major considerations are important when counseling patients with bladder cancer: First, the significance of a single tumor, multiple visible tumors, or multiple sites in the bladder which when biopsied are either obvious tumor or at least not typical in their appearance under the microscope (atypia). Single lesions denote that the bladder will be a "better actor" than the bladder with multiple lesions or multiple areas which while not discreetly cancer, are beginning to look more angry under the microscope. However, as two-thirds of patients with bladder cancer will recur, clearly even the patient with the single, small lesion will require follow-up once that lesion is eliminated.

Second, the appearance of the biopsies under the microscope gives us some idea how the patient's bladder is likely to behave. We score the tumor's appearance from 1 to 4, with 1 being almost like normal tissue and 4 being very angry and bizarre. It's not difficult to understand that the more angry and bizarre the tumor looks under the microscope, the more aggressive will be its behavior.

Probably the greatest advance in the treatment of bladder cancer in the last 10 years has come from the ability to use other testing upon the tissues than simply the subjective tissue appearance under the microscope to study and predict tumor behavior. These are all based upon the principle that as a cancer becomes more aggressive in its behavior, it loses certain structures on its surface and inside each cancer cell through a process called "de-differentiation". It is, if you will, an "undoing" of the differences which occur in the different cells during our maturation in the womb. The degree of de-differentiation (and it is a spectrum) allows us to predict those cancers

111

which are more likely to recur or spread, hopefully allowing us to be more aggressive in our treatments earlier to minimize a bad outcome for the patient with a more aggressive tumor.

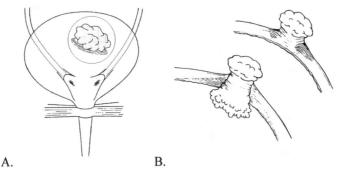

A.   B.
Figure 14-1: An invasive bladder cancer.

Third, the knowledge of the presence or absence of tumor rooted into the wall of the bladder allows us to better counsel the patients with bladder cancer (See Figure 14-1). Think of these tumors like the bush growing out in the front yard. If we wanted to get rid of it, we would not only clip it off at the ground level, but we would also use a spade to dig out the roots. In a manner of speaking, that's what a TURBT (transurethral resection of a bladder tumor, discussed later) is. With regards to the tissues, both the bush and the soil for possible roots (the tumor and fragments of the bladder wall at the tumor's base) are looked at microscopically. Not all tumors will extend into the wall of the bladder, but those that do require very vigorous treatment including possible removal of the entire bladder for cure.

Correlating grade (anger under the microscope) with stage (depth of invasion) allows us to give percentages and prognoses regarding the treatments of bladder cancer. In fact, most cancer counseling uses these two pieces of information, alone or in combination, to help patients to understand their disease and treatment options. Specifically with regards to bladder cancer, at the line between a grade 2 and a grade 3 tumor, the 50% likelihood of invasion is crossed, meaning that better than 50% of patients with a grade 3 or grade 4 tumor will have "sunken roots" and will require removal of the bladder entirely if they are to be cured (See Figure 14-2). Also during intravesicle chemotherapy, where chemical agents are placed into the bladder, retained generally for one hour, then urinated out) the changes either in the grade of the recurrent tumor or improvement in the other tests of "de-differentiation" may portend a better prognosis for the patient.

% Invasion

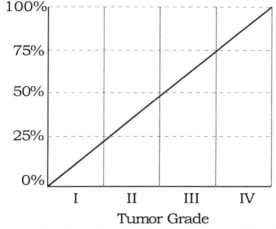

Tumor Grade

Figure 14-2: Graph relating bladder tumor grade and likelihood of invasion.

The tumor in the bladder is addressed by resecting or trimming the tumor out through a special cystoscope called the resectoscope. The instrument is the same as that used to trim the prostate gland for benign and utilizes electrical current. The tumor and a portion of the bladder at the base of the tumor is trimmed away. The tissue is retrieved from the bladder by a suction device, and a catheter is placed to drain the bladder for varying lengths of time depending upon the amount of post -operative bleeding. The tissue is then examined under the microscope to yield the above-described information.

Laser technology is also available for treatment of bladder cancer, instead of the standard resectoscope previously described which uses an electrical current. The laser probe operated operated through the cystoscope can reduce inflammation. The advantage of the laser is that the injury induced by the laser is more discreet, with less of a rim of inflammation (See Figure 14-3). Less inflamed tissue means that there will be less bladder irritation after the surgery and therefore fewer symptoms of urgency and frequency. Less inflammation also means less scarring.

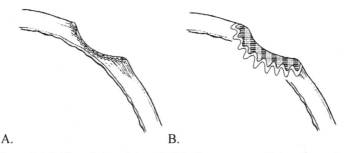

A.   B.

Figure 14-3: The cleaner injury left by laser energy (A.) compared with
       standard resection and cautery (B.).

For patients who experience frequent and numerous recurrences through the
years, scarring from numerous resections can actually compromise the
bladder's ability to stretch and serve as an adequate reservoir.

Disability following TURBT depends greatly upon the extent of resection
necessary and the healing ability of the patient. In principle, limitation of
activities is required to prevent bleeding from the resection site. Think of the
wound like a scrape. Squeeze a scrape, and it will bleed. Once a scrape has
been covered by a new skin lining, it will no longer bleed when squeezed.
You squeeze your bladder by any lifting or straining. In my practice for fairly
extensive resections, I will generally keep the patient home for a week. The
second week, the patient can be out in the car as a passenger, and during the
third week they can begin to drive. There is no heavy lifting or straining for 4
to 6 weeks with an additional 4 to 6 weeks before "full" activities are
resumed.

General followup for patients with bladder cancer includes cystoscopy every
3 months for 2 years (if there are no recurrences), followed by cystoscopy
every 6 months for 2 additional years, followed by annual cystoscopies for
the remainder of the patient's life. Usually annually , an IVP is performed as
the lining of the ureter and kidney also are of the same skin type (transitional
cell epithelium) as the bladder and are at risk to develop tumors. 10% of
bladder cancer patient's will develop cancer of the "upper tracts" (kidneys
and ureters). Some urologists also periodically send a voided urine specimen
for cytology, a special examination looking for cancer cells under the
microscope in the urine. Advocates of cytology feel this is a reasonable
substitute for some, but certainly not all, of the cystoscopies and IVP's
usually recommended. This is, however, a topic of debate among urologists.

The decision for or against additional treatment after resection depends upon the pathology report. Biopsies are performed in several different areas of the bladder even though these areas may not look particularly concerning for bladder cancer. This is called "bladder mapping", and is another useful tool in directing treatment. For the first tumor, single in number, of low grade, and with biopsies of the bladder away from the tumor showing no cancer or atypia, no additional treatment is recommended with the exception of surveillance cystoscopies as described above. If the tumor is high grade, if there are multiple tumors upon initial diagnosis, or if the biopsies away from the tumor show further cancer and/or atypia, then this denotes a bladder which is going to behave poorly if something is not done. Intravesicle chemotherapy is recommended in this setting.

With intravesicle chemotherapy, a chemical agent is placed into the bladder to be retained for approximately one hour. The patient is catheterized for its instillation, but can void the chemical out at home later. Generally, these are not begun until the bladder has healed from the resection. Several different agents are available, with differing treatment protocols and side effects.

If the bladder shows invasion into its wall (has sunken roots), the entire bladder must be removed for cure. The evaluation for any spread outside of the bladder is strikingly similar to that of the prostate. Bladder cancer can spread to the lymph nodes (filters) of the pelvis, the bones, the lungs, and the liver. Therefore, each of these is assessed by the "metastatic evaluation" prior to surgery in obtaining a CT scan of the abdomen and pelvis, bone scan, chest xray, and liver function tests which are included in a standard battery of blood tests. In males, the radical cystectomy includes removal of the bladder, prostate, seminal vesicles, and portions of the vas deferens which attach to the prostate. In females, the bladder, uterus, fallopian tubes, ovaries, and a portion of the vagina are all removed.

There are several options in the routing of the urine after radical cystectomy. The "gold standard" remains the ileal loop, in which a portion of the small bowel is isolated from the gastrointestinal stream, closed off at one end, attached to the ureters, and brought to the skin surface to be drained into a bag (Figure 14-4). Younger, healthier patients now allow us to convert pieces of intestine into reservoirs which can be drained by "in and out" catheterization techniques (a catheter is placed through a small stoma or opening on the skin, the reservoir is drained, and the catheter is removed). This obviously frees the patient of a bag, but there are more problems related to these procedures and a higher re-operation rate for complications or re-configuring.

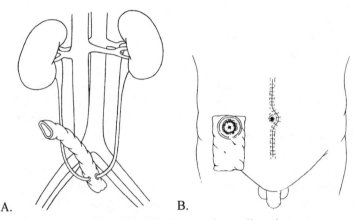

A. B.

Figure 14-4: The ileal loop urinary diversion.

Again, even after the bladder has been remove these patients require follow-up because of the risk of developing transitional cell cancers of the ureters or kidneys, the same cancer which afflicted their bladder.

Thus the bladder cancer patient in essence "marries" his or her urologist; for while the disease may be seemingly medically or surgically controlled, it requires surveillance for the remainder of the patient's life.

For more information write or call: American Cancer Society, 1599 Clifton Road, N.E., Atlanta, GA., 30329; (800) ACS-2345; or Cancer Information Service, National Cancer Institute, 550 N. Broadway, Room 307, Baltimore, MD., 21205; (800) 4-CANCER.

CHAPTER 15

TOILET TRAINING

Achieving toilet training.

Toilet training represents a very important milestone in child rearing, and signals an anxiously awaited change in lifestyle for the family: freedom from diapers and messes. The family's mobility and freedom for more unrestricted activities are now to be enjoyed. While a whole new set of experiences and problems await the parents, i.e. independence issues, the overall lifestyle of the family is improved. It is no wonder that many parents place undue pressures upon the child to toilet train and that toilet training itself may become an avenue for the surfacing of internal psychologic upset (for both parent and child) or of problematic family dynamics. Toilet training can become the weapon of the child for manipulation. Similarly, it may be or become a vicious tool used by a frustrated parent to demean or to manipulate the child. Conversely, if approached in a positive, nurturing way, toilet training can be among the most positive experiences for personal growth and confidence-building that a child can experience. The parents must have basic knowledge of what's occurring with their child in order to set reasonable expectations at appropriate stages of development. However, each child must have a tailored program for training--tailored by the parent for that child, for no one will know the child better than the parents. And what works well for one child will not necessarily work for another.

Two critical developmental milestones must be reached before a parent can be reasonably optimistic that toilet training can be accomplished. One is physiologic--having to do with bodily functions. The other is psychosociologic--having to do more with socialization skills.

Reaching the physiologic milestone means that the maturation of the central nervous system has occurred to suppress spontaneous evacuation of the bladder and bowel. Recall that the bladder wants to work all the time. The brain and central nervous system's job is to say "no". If there is no dampening or suppressing of this spontaneous activity, then fecal and urinary incontinence will occur all the time. Team this with a small bladder capacity, and it becomes obvious that the child needs to develop both more carrying capacity in the bladder and ample blocking of spontaneous contracting of the bladder. The size of a child's bladder can be estimated roughly by the equation:

$$\text{Capacity in ml.} = (\text{Age in years} + 2) \times 30$$

for example, a 2 year-old would have a bladder capacity of roughly 120 ml. Recall that there are 5 ml. in a teaspoon and 15 ml. in a tablespoon. Therefore, during the late second and into the third year of life, capacities are beginning to reach an attainable volume to serve as a reservoir to prevent wetting.

Second, the child's psychosociologic development must reach a point where urinary and fecal soiling are perceived by the child as unacceptable. In a non-traumatic way, the child must perceive accomplishing successful toilet training as an additional means (not sole means) of gaining social acceptance. But to place too much pressure on the child may not only be unfair physically, but also be a source of problems both immediate and delayed psychologically. Also psychosocially, the child must be mature enough to understand and seek rewards as a means of behavior modification.

If these two facets of development are achieved, toilet training can be easily accomplished. But if they have not been achieved, pathologic (problematic) patterns of urinating or defecating may occur which may be difficult to alter. One example we discussed is the learned behavior leading to Busy Little Girl (Boy) Syndrome in which the sphincters are tightened to such a degree to prevent leakage that they fail to relax entirely when urinating occurs. This leads to a hypertonic (high resting tone) bladder which feels as if it needs to go all the time or to repeated infection on the basis of incomplete emptying (See Chapter 9, Bladder Basics).

Most of the time the learned behavior of poor voiding is outgrown or resolves spontaneously, but on occasion we do see even older children and teenagers who have never experienced the joys of good urination or defecation. Let's call it the way it is: there are few free things in life which feel as good as a good whizz! Avoidance of confrontation over toilet training through the use of subtle manipulation will lead to more successful, uneventful toilet training. Be creative with rewards, but in the end the child will "call the signals" when ready.

CHAPTER 16

KIDNEY LUMPS

Cancer, cysts, and other lumps of the kidney.

This chapter details the benign (non-cancerous) and cancerous lumps (masses) of the kidney. Many of these conditions are discovered incidentally in the context of an evaluation being performed for another patient complaint or physician concern, i.e. a kidney mass is discovered during a CT Scan being performed because of nonspecific abdominal complaints. Usually they are discovered in an evaluation performed specifically for a urinary concern, i.e. microscopic or gross (visible) hematuria (blood in the urine).

ANATOMY AND FORMATION

Before a discussion of the specific conditions, a brief discussion of the upper urinary tract's anatomy and formation (embryology) would be helpful. In Figure 16-1, the "upper tracts" are seen to include the ureters (tubes which connect the bladder to each kidney), renal pelvis (the funnel-shaped receptacle which receives the urine from the different segments of the kidney), and the kidney itself including both the meat portion of the kidney (parenchyma) and the collecting system (the calyces and infundibuli which drain into the renal pelvis). The kidney filters the blood in its functional unit

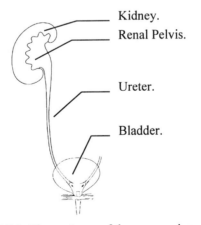

Kidney.
Renal Pelvis.

Ureter.

Bladder.

Figure 16-1: The anatomy of the upper urinary tract.

called the "nephron" and places the urine in a tube which then is expelled into the calyx through an opening on the papilla. The urine then travels down the infundibulum to the renal pelvis where it is propulsed down the ureter to the bladder. This is not a passive process, but rather one of active propulsion, much like intestinal contents are propulsed along. The ureters are muscular tubes. The direction of flow is from top to bottom for two reasons: urine is being constantly produce and sheer flow dynamics would dictate flow in this direction; secondly, the muscle of the renal pelvis and ureter is signaled to contract by an electrical impulse triggered and propagated from a location in the upper kidney through the renal pelvis and down the ureter to the bladder. The heart functions similarly in that an electrical impulse in the upper portion of the heart stimulates the smaller atrium to contract, squeezing the blood into the ventricles which then are stimulated to contract by the electrical impulse traveling in their muscular walls, thus propulsing the blood into the general circulation. The pressure created by peristalsis (coordinated contraction of the smooth-muscled ureter) is usually adequate to push urine along uneventfully; but with an obstruction, i.e. a kidney stone blocking the ureter, the pressure may rise quickly to levels which are interpreted as excruciatingly painful (See Chapter 17, Kidney Stones).

The best way to understand the kidney and ureter formation is to think of it like a flower (See Figure 16-2). Before you can have a blossom, you have to have a stem. The stem of the kidney take its origin from deep within the true pelvis--that is, our body's developing pelvis as distinguished from the kidney's pelvis which we previously described and illustrated.

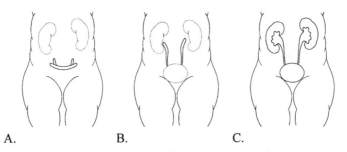

   A.   B.   C.

Figure 16-2: The development of the upper urinary tract.

Of course, although not completely formed yet, I find it easier to conceptualize if you think of our fully-developed body. The structure, for you Purists, is called the Mesonephric Duct System. This system at its bottom end is incorporated into the bladder. It "climbs" to the level of the kidney in much the same way a stem elongates as a solid column of cells.

When it reaches the area where cells have been coded to become the kidney (the Pronephros), the kidney develops like a blossom. The stem invests itself into the substance of the kidney by extensions of tissue which mold, shape, and become hollow thus forming the calyces, infundibuli, and renal pelvis of the kidney. And, the ureter hollows from its solid construction to a tubular structure to enable the urine to travel through it as the kidney begins to make early urine. This entire process is usually completed within the first 8 weeks of development in the mother's womb. Any failure of this formation, in any of its stages, may result in a problem in the development of normal architecture, a few of which are discussed below.

MULTICYSTIC KIDNEY

Broken down: multi (many), cystic (cysts), kidney; this is a problem in development diagnosed in newborns and infants generally by feeling an enlarged kidney on physical examination. The diagnosis is suspected by ultrasound, in which painless sound waves are directed at the kidney, revealing distorted anatomy of cysts in clustered like various-sized grapes on a stem (See Figure 16-3). The cause of Multicystic Kidney is thought to be a complete obstruction of the drainage of the kidney early in its formation so

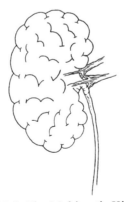

Figure 16-3: The Multicystic Kidney.

that when the kidney began to produce urine there was no drainage. The structures forming the ureter failed to hollow at all, completely blocking the

121

kidney's outlet. The back pressure and failure of drainage resulted in the dilation and stretching of the kidney as it formed and resulted in a functionless unit of cystic structures.

If the diagnosis remains unclear, a nuclear medicine study called a "renal scan" can reveal whether or not the cystic structure has function and the percentage it contributes to the patient's overall kidney function. Generally, Multicystic Kidneys are functionless. The decision to remove the Multicystic Kidney is depends upon whether or not the child shows any respiratory (lung function) limitation preventing adequate inspiration as a result of this sizeable (sometimes 8 to 10 times the normal kidney size) mass pushing on the diaphragm (the muscle which controls respiration). Similarly, if the mass pushes on the intestines or stomach to the point that feeding is compromised, that would be an indication to remove it. In the absence of complaints and with the certainty of diagnosis which our radiologic imaging can bring, these do not have to be removed. They will shrink over time or become smaller relative to the overall size of the patient as he or she grows. There is some debate in the urologic literature as to their malignant potential (to form cancer later), although most would agree that this is so remote that to remove all of these strictly on that basis only would not be indicated.

URETEROPELVIC JUNCTION OBSTRUCTION

Again broken down: uretero- (ureter), pelvic (pelvis), junction (joining), and obstruction (blockage), this is a blockage at the point where the renal pelvis of the kidney and ureter join (See Figure 16-4). This blockage either occurred

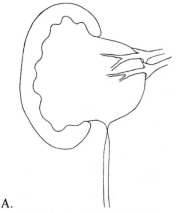

A.

Figure 16-4: The Ureteropelvic (UPJ) Obstruction.

at the same time as that which caused the Multicystic Kidney but was not as complete of blockage, or it occurred after the kidney was already past its developmental stage where its response to blockage would be the cystic kidney. What results is a kidney which has varying degrees of function plus anatomic distortion resulting in what can be massive amounts of urine housed in a stretched renal pelvis. The blockage is not only mechanical in the sense that urine has difficulty draining through the obstruction, but it is also physiologic, meaning that the electrical activity which is conducted down the ureter for normal peristalsis is impaired. In adults, an identical condition of mechanical blockage can occur as a result of a "crimping" of the ureter as it crosses occasionally present blood vessels which service the lower portion of the kidney.

These patients need not be infants. Children may present with nonspecific abdominal complaints, i.e. poor appetite or cramping, infection, or blood in the urine (either microscopic or gross). They may reveal visible blood in the urine with seemingly incidental trauma, i.e. a simple fall without serious injury, because this kidney is so tense with distension from urine that it is not as easily able to absorb the shock of a traumatic blow. This may be suspected as well by the finding of a mass in the loin or flank upon physical exam. In adults, occasionally we will see the patient with "Beer Drinker's Kidney". In this condition, the kidney becomes painful during states of aggressive hydration, i.e. with drinking of several glasses of fluids over a relatively short period of time. What occurs is that the blockage will allow only 2 ml. per minute to travel through it, for instance. During the period of hydration the patient may make 7 to 10 ml. per minute of urine in that kidney. Therefore, each minute results in a buildup of 5 to 8 ml. backed up into the kidney. If the stretched renal pelvis is able to hold 60 ml., in 7 to 12 minutes its capacity will be reached (5 ml. X 12 min.), and any additional volume placed into the renal pelvis will result in a raising of the pressure and the development of pain. The garden hose which has its internal pressure rise to very high levels between the house and where you've stepped on it provides a good example of this phenomena. Initially when first crimped, inflow exceeds outflow, and the hose fills to its limits Then the pressure rises as water is continually forced into the hose. With release of the hose, outflow will exceed inflow, and the hose will drain.

So it is with the kidneys. As the fluids coming on board are slowed or stopped, urine production will slow to a point where outflow exceeds production. The pelvis will drain, and the stretched pelvis will resume a more normal appearance. Thus, diagnosis is made with the patient well hydrated either by excessive drinking (of water, not beer!) or IV (intravenous) fluids, and then performing the xrays or scans.

The most accurate diagnostic test is called the retrograde pyelogram in which xray contrast or dye is injected backward up the ureter to the kidney by the urologist's placement of a small tube into the ureter through a cystoscopic look into the bladder. In children, this obviously would require an anesthetic and is frequently performed at the time of the surgical repair to insure the accuracy of the presumed diagnosis prior to surgery and to prevent the need for two anesthetics (one for the cystoscopy and one for the surgical repair). In adults, this can generally be performed with sedation and/or local anesthesia, but in many instances it is also performed simultaneously at the surgical repair in order to perform the evaluation and definitive surgery in one setting and to prevent the possibility of infecting the poorly drained space in the kidney thus causing a kidney infection, called pyelonephritis (See Infections of the Urinary Tract, Chapter 24).

The evaluation of a UPJ Obstruction also involves an assessment of the involved kidney's filtering function. If the kidney does not contribute more than 10% of the overall kidney function, it is probably not worth saving and will be removed. With less than 10% overall kidney function in the involved renal unit, it probably has been so damaged by the blockage that additional return of function cannot be expected. In addition, if the patient should experience a catastrophic loss of the good kidney on the opposite side, i.e. an accident, then even if a successful repair had been performed previously upon the involved kidney, that kidney still would not be sufficient to sustain the patient off dialysis. Therefore, it does not warrant salvage. The poorly draining kidney could continue to serve as a source of pain and/or infection, and therefore unless other medical reasons would preclude surgery, most urologists would recommend its removal.

The surgical removal of the kidney is performed through a variety of incisions but generally in a non-cancer condition it can be performed through the flank or side. The repair of the obstructed ureter is similarly approached. The segment is removed, if needed, the floppy pelvis of the kidney tailored to reduce its redundancy and dead space, and some form of drainage tube is placed, either internal for removal by cystoscopy later or external by a nephrostomy tube which is a tube through the side into the kidney (See Figure 16-5). All drainage tubes can be removed within a few days to few weeks, and the disability of the patient ranges from a few weeks to 3 months (kids always bounce back amazingly quickly). Follow-up studies, i.e. an IVP or nuclear medicine renal scan, are performed several weeks subsequent and

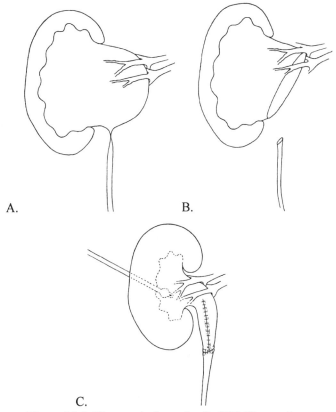

A.

B.

C.

Figure 16-5: The surgical repair of a UPJ Obstruction.

periodically thereafter for a few years. The long-term results for kidney salvage are excellent.

"DOUBLE" KIDNEY

If two stems ascend out of the pelvis on one side during early fetal development, a whole spectrum of anatomic variations may develop.(See Figure 16-6). Ten percent of the patients will have some "variation on a theme" of the upper urinary tracts, not all of which require surgical correction. If the timing is optimal in the development, two renal"segments" will develop, each of which functions normally and has its own collecting system (calyces, infundibuli, renal pelvis, and ureter). As each stem ascends, it touches cells

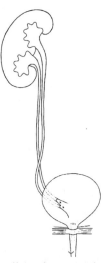

Figure 16-6: The duplicated upper urinary tract.

which are programed to develop into a kidney. Seldom are there two separate and complete kidneys on the same side of the body; but as the two kidneys mold and shape around their ureteral stem, they melt into a single kidney with some slight irregularity in contour, but with two draining ureters. If one stem comes up too early or too late, there will be aberration in the anatomy and function of that segment of the kidney, i.e. one segment may be normal and the other may be a nonfunctional cyst, or sac. Surgical reconstruction or removal is sometimes necessary based on the possibility of recurring infection or to optimize drainage to protect long-term renal function.

Two ureters on the same side is a critical discovery to make, particularly for a surgeon who may be contemplating surgery into that area, i.e. a bowel resection or a hysterectomy. Clear identification of the ureters at the time of an exploration prevents their inadvertent injury or transection (cutting totally in half) by a surgeon who has conscientiously identified one ureter in a patient who has two on that side. Frequently, for example, a gynecologist or general surgeon will order an IVP to visualize the urinary tract anatomy prior to an planned procedure.

Interestingly, recall that the lower end of the stem (Mesonephric Duct System) is incorporated into the bladder. Again, a whole host of anatomic variations can occur. Vesicoureteral reflux (See Figure 24-1in Infections of the Urinary Tract), in which urine is allowed to "yo-yo" back and forth between the kidney and bladder, is a result of an aberration in the incorporation of the ureter into the wall of the bladder. Ureterocoeles, balloon-like dilations at the end of the ureter, occur as a result of an incomplete hollowing of the bladder end of the tube. As urine is propulsed down the ureter by the newly formed kidney, the ureter from the bladder all the way to the kidney may balloon out and stretch yielding a condition called hydroureteronephrosis (hydro = water, + uretero = ureter, + nephros (kidney).

PELVIC OR "MISSING" KIDNEY

In some patients this complex development prevents the kidney from assuming its normal position up in the high flank. In some cases, the kidney(s) can be in the pelvis of the patient, usually at or near the branching of the iliac artery and vein (blood vessels) of the pelvis (See Figure 16-7).

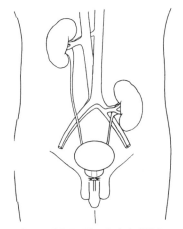

Figure 16-7: The Pelvic Kidney.

This anatomic variation is significant because this kidney may be in a position where it can cause pain, shed blood into the urine, or develop stones as a result of suboptimal drainage. Again, the importance of identifying this anatomic anomaly before any surgical procedure which brings a surgeon into this area is critical.

HORSESHOE KIDNEY

A very interesting anatomic configuration of aberrant kidney development is the kidney which is literally shaped like a horseshoe. The lower borders of each kidney has melted together. As a result of this, the kidney cannot rise up much out of the pelvis and it "hooks" around a sizeable blood vessel called the inferior mesenteric artery just like a well-thrown horseshoe hooks around its post (See Figure 16-8). This aberrant development also alters the drainage of the urine and frequently is partially blocked. Therefore, these patients, too, can have problems with pain, blood, and stones. Occasionally, this anatomic aberration requires surgical correction. Often, it is just a curiosity to the urologist and an important anatomical fact for the patient for potential future surgical procedures.

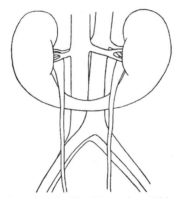

Figure 16-8: The Horseshoe Kidney.

KIDNEY CYSTS

A cyst is a fluid-filled sac. Kidney cysts are very common. If we are evaluating patients in their 50's, approximately 10 to 15% will have at least one renal (kidney) cyst. This figure rises by about 10% per decade. Patients with cysts are generally without symptoms. Occasionally they may cause problems either by becoming sizeable to the point that they cause pain by pushing on the surrounding structures, i.e. the intestines, or they may impair the drainage of the kidney yielding occasionally the appearance of a ureteropelvic junction (UPJ) obstruction (See previous discussion.).

Discovering a renal cyst requires certainty that the cyst is truly a "simple" cyst, meaning that it has no irregularity in its walls and it has no internal septations or dividing walls (See Figure 16-9). Either of these findings,

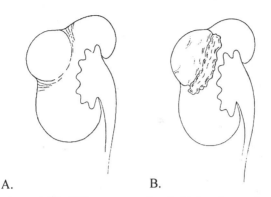

A.   B.

Figure 16-9: Kidney cysts: simple (A.) and complex (B.).

irregularity in the wall or septations, is associated with kidney cancer and would serve as an immediate indication to remove the kidney. The simplicity of a cyst is usually confirmed by a non-invasive test called the renal ultrasound, in which painless sound waves are echoed off of the kidney yielding an image of the kidney. No internal echoes are expected in a simple renal cyst, taking on the appearance in the study of a hollow ball.

Cysts require no treatment. Occasionally, if doubt remains regarding the diagnosis, a needle can be directed into the cyst utilizing CT Scan or ultrasound guidance. The fluid aspirated can be looked at under the microscope for cancer cells, and a medication can be placed into the cyst in to scar it closed. This is an outpatient procedure performed with local anesthesia, i.e. Lidocaine®. Cysts may very rarely require surgical exploration to rule-out cancer or for surgical excision (removal) or drainage.

INHERITED CYSTIC KIDNEY DISEASE

A rare occurrence is a stillborn child or a neonate who lives only very briefly due to a cystic disease of the kidneys which basically renders them functionless. The condition is called Infantile Polycystic Kidney Disease. Problems are suspected on the ultrasound performed upon the mother during pregnancy as the amount of amniotic fluid bathing the baby in the womb is dramatically less than we expect to see normally (oligohydramnios). The amniotic fluid is voided urine of the fetus. If the kidneys fail to make adequate urine, this will be noted on the ultrasound. Also, the kidneys of the fetus are dramatically enlarged, and these may also be seen on ultrasound prior to delivery. These kidneys look like a sponge with small, uniform-sized pores. Unfortunately, there is no treatment. The inheritance is called autosomal recessive, meaning that a gene would need to be donated by both the mother and father in order for it to occur. Neither parent would have kidney problems, although there may have been other kidney deaths in the families without the diagnosis being made.

A more common inherited cystic kidney disorder is called Adult Polycystic Kidney Disease. As opposed to that of infants, this is a dominant disorder, meaning at least ½ of the offspring of a patient could have the condition. All of these patients progress on to kidney failure and dialysis dependency. The problem here is that the condition is often not suspected until the patient is in the 40's or early 50's and ALREADY HAS HAD CHILDREN, who will also develop the disease in their 40's or 50's. Family counseling is extremely important for these patients and their families. These patients are suspected by changes in the blood tests for kidney function and the finding of extensive involvement of both kidneys with variable sized cysts. Frequently, these patients have blood pressure problems, pain, stones, or recurring kidney infections. Blood in the urine is common. Uncontrolled blood pressure problems or recurring infection may serve as indications to remove the kidneys prior to performing a kidney transplant (See Dialysis and Kidney Transplantation, Chapter 18). There is no cure nor are there any preventative measures for the affected patient, except family counseling to prevent pregnancies and future offspring who might be afflicted.

MEDULLARY SPONGE KIDNEY

This is a very common urologic anomaly limited to cysts in the central portion (medulla) of the kidney and dilated or stretched collecting tubules (the final portion of the nephron or unit of function in the kidney). This occurs in 1 in 5,000 of the general population and as many as 1 in 200 of patients with urologic disease. The small cysts are frequently filled with stones. Kidney function is usually good unless infections or stones cause complications. The most common complaints of patients are pain (colic) in 60%, hematuria (blood in the urine) in 30%, and stones in 40 to 50%. The prevention of problems and treatment for these patients are the same as those for any stone forming patient including the identification and correction of

130

the metabolic derangement and treatment for stones already formed (See Chapter 17, Kidney Stones).

KIDNEY CANCER

In children, a solid mass discovered in the kidney rarely occurs. A majority of children evaluated for a lump felt on physical exam will be either a Multicystic Kidney or a hydronephrosis (dilated renal pelvis and ureter) associated with a UPJ obstruction or possibly other congenital problems, i.e. reflux (See Chapter 9, Bladder Basics) or posterior urethral valves--a blockage of the urethra in which leaflets of tissue billow like wind in a sail during urination and obstruct the urinary outflow. If, during the evaluation a solid mass is diagnosed, particularly in the 2-to-3 year old, Wilm's Tumor is possible. This is an extremely aggressive cancer which requires aggressive surgical excision and additional treatment frequently with chemotherapy and/or radiation. Even with such biologic behavior, 5-year survival figures for children with Wilm's Tumor now exceed 80%, that is, 80% of these children will live 5 years or longer.

Adults are suspected to have kidney cancer with blood in the urine (See Chapter 14, Blood in the Urine and Bladder Cancer) as 50% of kidney cancers will be associated with hematuria. 50% will have a mass which is detected on physical exam. 50% will have pain. The classic triad of pain, hematuria, and flank mass are rarely found together in the same patient. With hematuria, generally the routine evaluation will be performed including an IVP and cystoscopy. An anatomical distortion will usually be apparent on IVP. Cystoscopy is still indicated to eliminate another process in the bladder, i.e. a bladder cancer. Recall that these patients are also in the age group to have bladder or prostate cancers. Approximately 11,000 new cases were newly diagnosed and treated with cancer of the kidney in 1993, accounting for approximately 3% of all adult malignancies.

Renal cell cancer is a very strange tumor. It can be a great imitator of other medical conditions in ways which we don't entirely understand. These are called a paraneoplastic syndromes. For example, strange and unusual fevers may be the patient's primary complaint, or erratic blood pressures, alterations in some of the patients' blood chemistries, liver problems, or blood count disorders. Weight loss, fatigue, and abnormal liver studies on blood testing, all yield a poor prognosis.

Renal cell cancers spread to the lymph nodes around the kidneys, the bone, the liver, and the lungs. Prior to any surgical removal, these areas assessed with CT Scan, bone scan, chest xray, and blood tests to assess liver function. Additional studies are performed to assure that the patient's opposite, good kidney will be capable of providing adequate filtration function (called the "clearance") to prevent dialysis. This usually involves the collection of the urine for 24 hours and performing clearance studies. That number is then roughly halved to yield the output of the good kidney. A"ballpark" estimate of clearance is to take 100 divided by the serum creatinine (a blood test). For instance, a healthy patient with no kidney disease would have a creatinine of 0.8, for instance; therefore, the clearance would be 125 ml./min. (= 100/ 0.8). If that number is greater than 20 ml./min., the patient has adequate function. Between 10 to 20 ml./min., there probably is adequate function, but little or no reserve. Less than 10 ml./min. will not be sufficient to sustain the patient off of dialysis. While a cancer-curing operation would certainly not be withheld, the possibility of permanent dialysis would require discussion prior to the nephrectomy. Assuming that there is no evidence of spread outside of the kidney to distant sites, additional studies may be necessary to look at the major blood vessels draining the kidney, as occasionally the tumor may extend as a tongue of tissue into the main renal vein Rarely, this column of tumor may extend all the way to the heart.

The surgery for removal, called a radical nephrectomy (nephros = kidney, + ectomy = removal) is usually performed through an incision which parallels the lower border of the rib cage. Radical nephrectomy differs from the simple nephrectomy described above. In the radical nephrectomy, the kidney and its surrounding structures are removed (See Figure 16-10). Think of the

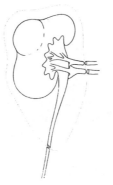

Figure 16-10: The radical nephrectomy for kidney cancer.

kidney like a letter. The letter sits in an envelope of tissue called Gerota's fascia. With a simple nephrectomy, we open the envelope and take out the letter. With a radical nephrectomy, the letter is removed with the envelope never opened. The blood vessels are tied off as they enter and exit the envelope, and the kidney is removed. This minimizes the risk of tumor "spill" during the operation. The "complete" disability time is approximately 6 weeks, followed by 6 additional weeks of partial disability depending upon the patient's work type.

Survivals to 5 years of 70% are expected if the tumor is confined to the kidney, meaning 70% of individuals with disease confined to the kidney will survive for 5 years or greater. For limited spread outside of the kidney, 35 to 50% 5 year survivals are expected. For patients with spread to distant sites at the time of presentation, less than 10% will survive 2 years, therefore no surgery is offered unless contemplated to improve the patient's lifestyle, i.e. to lessen pain from the tumor or to alleviate bleeding. Renal cell carcinoma has not shown much response to additional treatments with chemotherapy or radiation. Several investigational studies are proceeding, especially in the arena of immunotherapy, in which our body's immune system is activated to combat the cancer.

An additional type of tumor in the kidney and ureter is one similar to bladder cancer. The hollow portion of the kidney (calyces, infundibuli, renal pelvis, and ureter) is lined by the same skin lining as that of the bladder, called transitional cell epithelium. Therefore, cancers similar to bladder cancer can occur at these sites as well.These tumors account for only 7% of all kidney cancers, yet they are also extremely aggressive tumors. Fortunately, they do tend to present with much smaller tumors as they bleed readily into the urine.

If a renal cell cancer is located on the periphery of the kidney, even if it bleeds, it will not be suspected as the blood will often not be visible in the urine. However, with transitional cell tumors of the renal pelvis and ureter, blood is seen earlier (See Figure 16-11). The evaluation again involves an IVP and cystoscopy. The IVP will lead to suspicion of the diagnosis. A retrograde pyelogram may also be performed. The tumor may be "brushed" by a small tube with a brush on the end placed by cystoscopy up to the site suspected and rubbed against the tumor. The cells obtained on the brush are viewed under the microscope to yield the diagnosis. With great advances in instrumentation, urologists now have the technical capability to proceed up the ureter with special scopes to view the tumor directly (ureteroscopy), perform biopsies, and possibly even destroy the tumor completely, as with

133

bladder tumors, thus precluding the need to remove the entire kidney (in selected cases). If ureteroscopy cannot be performed for technical reasons or

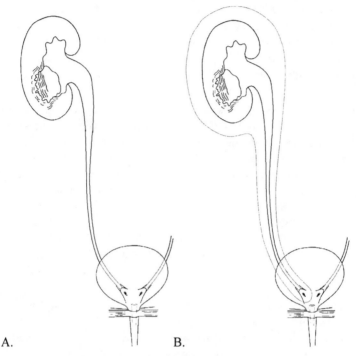

A.   B.

Figure 16-11: The transitional cell kidney cancer.

concerns regarding complete elimination of disease, then complete removal of the kidney, ureter, and a ring of bladder surrounding the ureteral meatus (the opening into the bladder of the ureter) is indicated.

These patients will need continued surveillance just like bladder cancer patients (See Chapter 14, Blood in the Urine and Bladder Cancer) as between 15 and 50% will go on to subsequently have bladder cancer. Survivals range from 70 to 100% for disease limited to the most shallow skin layer, 40 to 50% if roots have been sunk partially through the underlying muscle layer of the ureter or renal pelvis, and less than 10% for tumors which have invaded full thickness or are spread to distant sites. If the disease is not surgically cured, additional treatments are available with both chemotherapy and radiation therapy.

SUMMARY

In summary, our ability to image by various radiologic procedures (nuclear scans, ultrasound, IVP, CT Scan, and retrograde pyelography) makes exploration for a kidney or ureteral mass without a diagnosis and full understanding of extent of disease an extremely unusual case. Radiologic procedures have lead to the diagnosis in an unsuspecting setting of up to 10% of kidney cancers by discovery through studies performed for other diagnoses, the so called "incidental" discovery. The urologic evaluation, though not "knee-jerk", relies upon its "gold standard": the IVP and cystoscopy. Early discovery provides the greatest outlook for a favorable outcome. Any concern regarding weight loss, early satiety, mass in the abdomen, pain in the loin or flank, or blood in the urine should prompt an immediate visit to a physician's office.

CHAPTER 17, SECTION A

KIDNEY STONES: CAUSES

All aspects of kidney stone disease.

No area of urology, and perhaps of medicine in general, exemplifies better the blending of technological advances with medical knowledge to provide dramatic improvements in patient care. Kidney stones account for one of approximately every 750 hospital admissions per year and afflict thousands of patients annually. Up to 70% of those will be "repeat offenders" if no preventative measures are taken. The problem is generally a younger persons' disorder, striking between the ages of 20 to 45 years with males 2 to 3 times more commonly afflicted than females and Caucasians 3 to 4 times more likely to experience than Negroes. Employers and insurers are interested in the newer treatments particularly as they are less morbid (meaning less associated with long hospitalizations and time of disability after) and they are more preventative (in that 80% or so of stone formers have an identifiable metabolic or anatomic factor which predisposes them to recurrence).

Upon completion of the three sections of this chapter, the reader should be able to understand in a general sense how stones form, upon formation how they cause problems, the different approaches to treatment of stones, and finally, some general understanding of prevention.

STONE FORMATION

To understand how stones form, think of adding sugar to a glass of water (See Figure 17-1). If just the right amount of sugar (let's say one teaspoon) is added to a drinking glass of water, the entire teaspoon of sugar will stay suspended in the water after stirring. Add more sugar to the same glass, and the sugar will become too saturated to be suspended, and it will crystallize even while stirring and settle to the bottom of the glass when stirring has stopped. Add the same-sized teaspoon of sugar to a shot glass of water, and it will immediately crystallize out and settle to the bottom of the glass. The final experiment goes back to our original concoction, in which sugar and water volume are in perfect balance to keep the sugar suspended. Let this glass sit on the counter overnight, and even eliminate the factor of evaporation and assume that no volume is lost. In the morning when you

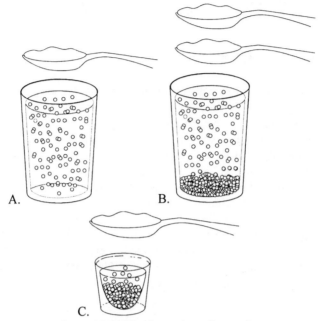

Figure 17-1: The formation of crystals.

return, you will find a significant portion of the sugar crystallized at the bottom of the glass.

Stones form in just this way: Let's say that CHEMICAL X, whether it be calcium, uric acid, oxalate, cysteine, or magnesium ammonium phosphate (the most common chemicals yielding stone formation), is the most common stone forming chemical. In most of us, X can be washed away because we neither make too much of it nor are we short in making adequate urine volumes to keep it suspended until we can eliminate it. However, some of us make too much CHEMICAL X, through errors in our metabolism. The volume of fluids we ingest and therefore the urine we make just isn't adequate to keep all of CHEMICAL X suspended, and therefore it crystallizes--much like when we added additional sugar to our drinking glass of water. If we measure the amount of CHEMICAL X which we place in our urine in 24 hours, we will find it to be very high.

If on the other hand we have no metabolic problem, we might find that our amount of CHEMICAL X in the urine for a 24-hour period is normal. If our volume of urine, though, was extremely low, that is, our urine would be extremely concentrated, we would form crystals like the teaspoon of sugar placed in the shot glass.

If, our metabolism and fluid balance were just right, but we had an anatomic blockage in the kidney preventing prompt and complete drainage of the urine as it was being made, crystals could form much the same as the normal drinking glass which sat on the counter overnight.

Two final slightly more complex scenarios probably depict most stone formers: The 24-hour value for CHEMICAL X is normal, and the volume of urine made in a 24-hour period also looks adequate, yet stones still form. There are probably periods of dehydration during which the urine is very concentrated, i.e. the rough carpenter working all day out in the very hot sun, but who drinks more than enough fluids in the evening to replenish his system and to make his 24-hour values look good. His crystals form during the day, when he's dry. Alternatively, stone formation with overall normal values could be exemplified by a eating that huge meal at our favorite restaurant. Our digestive system goes to work barraging our system with CHEMICAL X, perhaps supersaturating us for a short period of time and overwhelming the ability of the volume of urine being made at that time to keep CHEMICAL X suspended. For a short period of time crystals are again produced, even though measurement of both CHEMICAL X and the volume of urine made for the 24-hours in question may be normal. Both of these slightly more complex scenarios demonstrate that metabolism is a dynamic process. Seldom is our body in any of its processes like an assembly line working at the same pace all day, performing its function at exactly the same rate or with exactly the same result.

Now we have some crystals formed, but how do we end up with stones? Many times we will not--the crystals will be passed in total silence, only to be detected if we were to have a microscopic examination of the urine (urinalysis). Under the microscope crystals are beautiful, taking on very characteristic geometric shapes depending upon what type of chemical is crystallizing, i.e. hexagons for calcium oxalate, octagons for a cysteine, "coffin lids" for magnesium ammonium phospate (struvite). Even though the patient may not have had any stone passages or show any new or enlarged stones on xray, the presence of crystals in the urine would indicate the potential for active stone formation and the need for better control to prevent stone formation.

Crystals bunch together and form stones like LEGOS® fitting together. They form a lattice. Once this process is initiated, a nidus or center forms, around which a small stone develops--one not even large enough to yet be seen on xray. This process usually occurs attached to the wall of the kidney tubule or collecting system, much like the residue which builds over time in a pipe. With each shower of new crystals formed in any manner previously described, new layers of additional crystals are added to our nidus eventually yielding a large enough stone to become "clinically significant" (translation: It can hurt if it moves!). The stone eventually becomes "heavy" enough that it tears off from its attachments to the wall of the kidney's lining, much like a cluster of branches you've watched collect at the edge of a briskly flowing stream. Eventually, as more debris is added, the cluster tears free and flows on down the stream until it again becomes snagged at some other narrowed or shallow point. It is at these snag points that stones can cause some very uncomfortable times for patients. In the formation process and until a stone moves into a position that it causes a blockage, it will be housed silently. Stones in and of themselves are painless--it's the body's response to their becoming lodged in an attempt to be passed that causes pain.

SYMPTOMS OF STONE DISEASE

Let's review briefly some pertinent anatomy in order to understand how stones cause problems. The kidney filters the blood to produce urine. This is a very complex process, with each type of chemical being handled in a slightly different manner. Physicians who specialize in diseases intrinsic to the kidney are called nephrologists (nephros: kidney; + ologist: student of). They also run patient dialysis when the kidneys fail, and filtration is performed by a machine (See Chapter 18, Kidney Transplantation and Dialysis).

The units of the kidney performing the filtration are called the nephrons (See Figure 17-2). Each kidney has approximately one million nephrons. Each has a tuft where the blood comes in and is forced through a very convoluted knot of tiny vessels and then a tube through which the filtrate (the fluid filtered out of the blood) travels and is acted upon. As the blood exits the tuft (called the glomerulus) to return to the general circulation, the filtered portion is placed

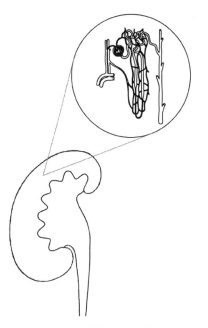

Figure 17-2: The kidney and its nephron.

into the long tube. During its passage, a number of very complex processes occur which allow the body to retrieve from the filtrate those things which it wishes to salvage and return into the circulation (Think of it as a form of "recycling"). In general then, much kidney disease is not that the kidney couldn't filter, but that it fails to salvage those things, i.e. certain proteins, salts, and other necessary chemicals, which it should to keep metabolism in good balance.

The filtered fluid in its final stages of passage through the nephron is concentrated--this process is performed as the body recognizes its need to maintain good body fluid balance. If you've been out working in the yard all afternoon and your fluid status is low, your kidneys will retrieve most of the fluid back into the system, making very concentrated urine likely to form stones (See above). If on the other hand, you've been watching the triple-header of NFL football all Sunday afternoon with your right hand tightly wrapped around your favorite brew, then you can expect your urine to be dilute (and your waist size to be larger than it should be!).

The central nidus of stone formation frequently will become lodged in the most terminal portions of the nephron called the collecting duct, in an environment which finds the urine most concentrated. If a stone forms in this location, it may become large enough to rupture into the collecting system, yielding varying degrees of pain and/or blood.

The final passage within the kidney tubule normally finds the urine being purged into the "collecting system" of the kidney. Think of the kidney as having a "meat" portion where all the nephrons are and a hollow central portion like a funnel (See Figure 17-2). The main funnel is called the renal pelvis, but actually it is serviced by a number of additional funnels called calyces (calyx: chalice or cup), draining the top, middle, and bottom of the kidney. It is into each of theses calyces that the nephrons drain through spigots called a papillae (papilla: mound). A stone may have erupted from the collecting duct but may be too large to fit through the neck, called an infundibulum, and therefore becomes trapped--periodically causing pain as it drops like a ball-valve into position to block that portion of the kidney, continuously adding crystals to its volume.

The stone may have been small enough to fit through the infundibulum, or perhaps it was forced through as the pressure behind the stone from the continued urine production eventually overcame the resistance of the neck holding it in place, much like forcing your way through a door with someone on the other side trying to hold it closed. It is now in the largest funnel, the renal pelvis. There it may be silently housed, rolling around, adding crystalline growth to its edges like a snowball enlarging as it rolls down a hill. It may cause severe pain as it periodically falls into a position to block the flow of urine down the ureter (the tube connecting the kidney to the bladder).

The ureter, a muscular tube, serves not just as a passive conduit to carry the urine from the kidney to the bladder, but also actively pushes the urine through, just like the intestines "move" their contents along. For kidney stones, there are three particular areas of narrowing of the ureter which limit passage (See Figure 17-3). First, previously described, the junction of the renal pelvis and the ureter is a narrow point. Second, as each ureter courses over the pelvic brim and dives into the deep pelvis, it must cross the large blood vessel (called the iliac artery) which splits off of the aorta (our bodies' largest blood vessel) and travels to each leg. This bump as the ureter courses over this vessel sometimes snags the stone. Finally, as the ureter joins with the bladder, the point of tightest constriction is met. The junction is not like a

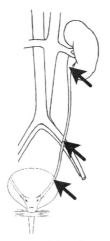

Figure 17-3: The ureter and locations of narrowing.

pipe coming through a wall at a right angle, with only the thickness of the wall as the length of constriction. Rather, the ureter enters through the bladder obliquely (at an angle) in order to prevent urine from going back to the kidney as the pressure rises in the bladder during urination (See Figure 24-1 in Chapter 24, Infections of the Urinary Tract).

The best illustration, as in Figure 24-1, of this anatomical relationship is to hold your hand upright with all fingers and the thumb aligned and together straight. A pencil held at a right angle and held between the middle and ring finger will traverse only the thickness of the fingers. However, a pencil angled will traverse the thickness of the fingers in a distance equal to or longer than the fingers themselves. This oblique course means that the constriction is over a longer length of the ureter and is more likely to prevent spontaneous passage of the stone.

The character and location of the pain can give clue to the location of the stone and the level of obstruction. Kidney and upper ureteral pain, that is near the kidney, typically can be referred to the testicle in the male and the labia of the female. This occurs because of the shared nerves to these areas and the brain's inability to decipher the difference between the exact anatomic origin of the incoming messages. We will discuss the origin of the testicles as near that of the kidneys in Chapter 21 (Male Self Examination and Testes Cancer). As the stone moves down the ureter, the pain becomes more loin or flank, than groin. The final stages of pain are bladder pain as the stone is forced through the tunnel in which the ureter is housed in the wall of the bladder. Symptoms mimic the tremendous urge to urinate despite emptying only a small amount--again the brain only hears one message from the bladder ("I've got to go!"), whether it be on the basis of being full or being fooled by the tremendous irritation of the stone's passage.

The two holes created as the ureters empty into the bladder, one on each side, form 2 of the 3 points of a triangle on the floor of the bladder (See Bladder Basics, Figure 9-3). The third point is the bladder neck, through which the urine exits to be emptied. This triangle, called the trigone, contains the highest concentration of nerves which signal the brain. With stone passage, at least a portion of this surface will be tremendously inflamed, yielding symptoms. Occasionally, again because of a shared relationship in their embryology, the last stage of pain will be associated with shooting pain to the tip of the penis or to the opening of the female urethra. The bladder symptoms then usually characterize the final stages of stone passage. Remember as well that crystals too, while considerably smaller, can cause pain as they scour the lining of the kidney, ureter, or bladder in their descent. Generally speaking, if a kidney stone has successfully made it into the bladder, it will pass through urination.

Primary bladder stones, that is, stones which originate in the bladder, usually form on the basis of either some form of obstruction, i.e. an older gentleman with incomplete bladder emptying from prostate enlargement, or they form because of some primary bladder structural problem, i.e. a pouch or dog ear on the bladder (diverticulum) which never is completely emptied when the bladder purges itself. Either process here is like the normal drinking glass containing CHEMICAL X which sat overnight; in other words, urinary stasis will provide the opportunity for stone formation. Often these stones will be multiple and quite sizable--the largest I've seen was slightly larger than a baseball, obviously requiring surgical removal.

In summary, stones cause pain as they become ensnared. They cause irritation at that point, causing the tissues to inflame, swell, and entrap the stone even tighter. All the while, urine continues to be manufactured by the kidney and is placed in the renal pelvis and ureter. With obstructed outflow, the pressure rises between the kidney and the level of the obstructing stone, much like stepping on a hose and partially crimping it. Between your foot and the spigot at the house, the pressure rises. Pressure is perceived as painful--and again, the level to which the pressure occurs yields characteristic symptoms for the patient.

If the pressure is high enough and prolonged, two interesting phenomena occur, either of which or both acting in concert may alleviate the pain even though the stone continues to remain in its obstructing position. The pressure may cause a leak and the urine will become reabsorbed back into the system directly into the bloodstream or into the lymphatic system. The point of maximal weakness where this is most likely to occur is in the kidney around each of the papillae (See Figure 17-2). Additionally, through a process called accommodation, constant messages sent back to the brain, i.e. a continuously painful process, over time fail to be consciously perceived. Consider your wristwatch. When you first put your watch on you notice it. Over time, you don't feel it, even though the nerves compressed by the watchband continue to send their messages back to the brain. The danger with the asymptomatic obstruction is that the damage to the kidney continues. With 100% obstruction for approximately 6 weeks or longer, a significant and irreparable damage to the kidney can occur. With partial obstruction, the process will take longer. Therefore, one indication to surgically treat an asymptomatic stone is a concern that the patient will not be compliant, i.e. not return after a reasonable time of conservative management to have the stone removed, and therefore will suffer injury or even loss of a kidney.

The damage from obstruction will first affect the ability of the kidney to concentrate the urine--the patient's fluid requirements may be much greater because the kidney will not be effective at salvaging fluid to maintain good fluid balance. Translation: the patient will have to drink much more because they'll be urinating a whole lot more. Second, the kidney will lose its ability to acidify the urine, that is, to get rid of the acids created in the body's many and complex chemical reactions. Translation: the patient will feel ill and may note dramatic changes in respirations because the lungs, through a sequence of very complicated metabolic reactions, will attempt to blow off the acid from the system. Finally, the kidney's ability to filter will be compromised, and there will be total disarray in the chemical and fluid balance. These endpoints will seldom be reached clinically because the generally healthy patient will have another kidney upon which to rely and to pick up the slack. In the patient with compromised kidney function for other reasons, the loss of a renal unit may be significant. But the involved kidney may be silently lost.

In the following sections, we will continue our discussion of stone disease by covering the treatment of and prevention of urinary calculi (kidney stones).

CHAPTER 17, SECTION B

KIDNEY STONES: TREATMENT

The treatment of urinary stones truly demonstrates the blend of physician skill, technological advances, and patient compliance (cooperation). As with most diseases in the surgical discipline, the judgment of when and how to intervene significantly predicts outcome. Fantastic instruments used incorrectly can have disastrous results; similarly, "mechanical breakdown" of equipment can render an extremely disappointing result even with the most skillful surgeon.

The treatment of kidney stones can be divided into three major categories: open surgical, endoscopic (performed through telescopes), and extracorporeal lithotripsy, or ESWL®, (machinery which pulverizes stones without surgery and makes fragment passage more possible). Deciding which treatment to use, alone or in combination, is part of the arduous six-year training to become a urologist and involves choice of instrumentation or technique based upon the likely type of stone, its anatomic location, and the availability of the technology.

Surgery is the "gold standard" against which all other techniques must be compared, not only because it is historically the oldest of treatments, but also because it has the highest success rates. Stones were uniformly operated upon if they were anatomically not likely to pass, were multiple and sizable, or if there was an anatomic problem which clearly required simultaneous correction at the same surgical setting to prevent future stone formation. For example, if the neck of the funnel connecting the kidney to the ureter (the ureteropelvic junction) is too tight, creating a blockage and stagnation of urine resulting in stone formation, then in addition to removal of the stone this area should be corrected of its blockage. The two most common settings in which surgery is still utilized is the correction of such an anatomic problem or if less invasive procedures, i.e. an endoscopic instrumentation or ESWL®, have failed.

Endoscopic retrieval of stones was, until the last few years, relegated to stones which had traversed to near the junction of the ureter with the bladder where they could be retrieved though the use of various wires and baskets. With the advent of fiberoptic scopes, teamed with flexible instruments and working tools, literally the entire urinary tract can be approached endoscopically--either through access through the bladder and up the ureter in a "retrograde" fashion or, less commonly, through a tract or access created to the kidney (percutaneous or puncture through the skin technique) which allows entrance to the kidney and the ureter from above in an "antegrade" fashion. The most recent addition endoscopically has been the utilization of laser energy carried through small wires or probes which fit easily through the scopes and allow the fracturing of a sizable stone into more easily retrievable smaller fragments.

Extracorporeal Shock Wave Lithotripsy, or ESWL®, is truly a development of Nobel Prize proportions. This treatment allows for outpatient or short hospital stay settings for stones which previously required several hospital days, painful surgery, and prolonged periods of disability. Typically the treatments are done under regional anesthesia (for example, epidural anesthesia with the addition of sedation), require considerably less than an hour to perform, and the patients have very short periods of disability, if any at all. With newer machines, no anesthesia or sedation may be possible. Success rates for a relatively uncomplicated stone of reasonable size (say a half inch or less) range in the 92 to 95% success rate for one treatment. Again, a major consideration in the success of the treatment is the judgment as to whether or not this treatment should be used at all. If our patient above, with the blockage preventing good drainage of the kidney, had lithotripsy without correction of the blockage, its highly likely that the treatment would not be successful because the fragments would be unable to drain would serve as niduses for future stones to form. The patient would end up with several stones rather than the single stone with which he or she started.

How does ESWL® work? (See Figure 17-4). Think of the energy created to fracture the stone as similar to the energy carried in a wave in a pond of water. When you drop a pebble on the pond, the instant the pebble strikes the surface it compresses the water molecules under it. They then unleash this energy in all directions in the form of a mechanical shock wave or ripple. The energy we create during lithotripsy is by an electrical shock wave, a very powerful electrical shock wave in the range of 18,000 to 24,000 volts. The electrical shock created in an immersed spark plug compresses the water molecules in the spark gap. The compressed water molecules then release their wave. The wave travels in all directions, but in ESWL®, it is released inside of a bowl (actually an ellipsoid, or half of an ellipse). The bowl then serves to reflect and aim the shock wave. This occurs in much the same way

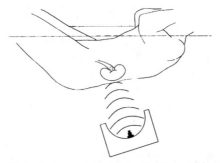

Figure 17-4: Extracorporeal Shock Wave Lithotripsy®.

as a wave would be reflected as it traveled across a quiet pond to a boulder protruding out of the water. The mathematics of this process (an ellipsoid for all of you math whizzes) are such that all the energy is directed to one point, which is precisely where the patient is positioned to allow the stone to occupy that point. This movement of the patient is performed utilizing xray and is reassessed during the treatment so that adjustment can be made to ensure optimal treatment. The shock wave fractures the stone along crystalline lattice lines. Each additional shock wave triggered by the patient's EKG (heart tracing) fractures the stone more and more. As an aside, the R wave of the EKG is used, interestingly, because this is the time when the heart is most resistant to any outside electrical activity, thus preventing any irregular heart beats caused by the electrical energy used for the treatment.

As one fragment becomes two, then four, and so on the shock wave is "echoed" back and forth between the fragments allowing a better degree of pulverization. Stones tightly packed in an anatomic location, i.e. a stones lodged tightly in the ureter, are not as likely to be well pulverized as a "loose" stones up in the kidney. The ultimate goal is the complete disintegration of a stone into powder with the consistency of sand which can be passed uneventfully and within a few weeks after treatment.

Does the presence of a stone mandate that it be treated? Absolutely not! Because our treatments have improved and can be less invasive, less morbid, and less costly does not dictate that all stones be treated. One would not argue with the decision to treat the patient with pain or with an obstructed kidney--be it painful or not. But the 63 year-old, asymptomatic female with a 4 mm (roughly 1/6th of an inch) located in a calyx does not need to be treated. It is quite possible that the stone has been present for quite some time and is unlikely to ever cause problems. She can easily be observed with an occasional xray to ensure that no new stones have formed or that the known stone has not enlarged. That same stone in a 43 year-old commercial pilot will require treatment however, as he is "grounded" until he is stone free. So each treatment must be custom-tailored to the patient.

A word regarding comparative cost of these various treatments is in order. Let's use as our example a 1-inch kidney stone with no other patient conditions. Considering now only the surgical and hospital charges, the open surgical procedure is assigned $X for the charges. The percutaneous stone procedure would incur charges of $X/2, or roughly one-half of the open charges. ESWL® charges would be $X/4, or roughly one-fourth of the charges when compared to the "gold standard" open surgical procedure.

Add on top of this savings is the very important employer consideration of disability time. Disability eliminates a potentially valuable employee from the workplace while at the same time also siphons additional funds from the employer's financial resources. An open surgical procedure routinely has "complete" disability time of nearly 6 weeks, with an additional 6 weeks of "partial" disability dependent upon the type of work performed, i.e. an accountant would be expected to return to full productivity sooner than a cement truck driver. Endoscopic procedures routinely have total disability time of less than 3 weeks, and with ESWL® the time is further reduced to routinely 3 to 5 days at most.

Together then, the reduced hospital costs and the reduced disability time have lessened the financial burden of benefits programs for the treatment of **any given patient** with stone disease. However, the "total bill" for **all patients** with stone disease has not appreciably dropped because many patients are being treated with ESWL® who otherwise would **not** have been treated by more traditional means, i.e. "silent" or small stones, patients with medical conditions which might prove prohibitive for open surgical procedures, or patients who previously on the basis of age or unlikelihood to add to or form other stones were previously not counseled to undergo treatment by surgery. In part there is some blame to bear by urologists who fail to use those same stringent criteria which we would employ in selecting a patient elgible for more traditional means of surgical treatment when considering ESWL®.

CHAPTER 17, SECTION C

KIDNEY STONES: PREVENTION

The two best ways to prevent any problem are to identify the problem clearly and to identify those at risk for that problem. For a stone former, the best prevention first involves knowing what type of stone has formed and identifying those factors which may lead to the formation of other stones. There should also be concern for any immediate family member (blood relative). For instance, a urinalysis should become a regular part of a physical exam and check for family members of known stone-formers. Crystals detected in one of these individuals may lead to the discovery by further evaluation, i.e. a KUB (single xray of the abdomen without dye to show the kidney, ureters and bladder), of a totally silent stone leading to treatment before problems ensue. By further metabolic evaluation, direct treatment preventing any enlargement of the existing stone or formation of new stones can be instituted.

Collecting a stone for analysis is critical to identify the problem. Sounds obvious and simple, right? However, nearly one-third of stones passed in the hospital are lost or discarded, and these are patients under professional care for this very reason! Once analyzed the stone will most likely return as below:

Calcium oxalate	45%
Calcium phosphate	30%
Uric acid	15%
Magnesium ammonium phosphate	10%
(Struvite)	
Cystine	<1%

The evaluation of the calcium stone former can be explained by referring to the following flow diagram (Figure 17-5). The evaluation is really quite simple for the patient to complete. The patient goes to the lab, at which time a sample of blood is taken for calcium and uric acid, and a container is given for collection of urine for 24 hours. The container is returned upon completion of the 24-hour urine collection and a second sample of blood is taken for the same chemical constituents. These will allow us 80% accuracy in earmarking and treating any calcium stone former.

150

Before we discuss the results, a word on 24 hour urine collections. Physicians have been frustrated (as well as patients) by an inaccurate or incomplete collection by patients usually as a result of misunderstood directions. Let me take a few moments and explain it.

First, a 24-hour collection done at home requires some forethought because it must be done through a significant period of time when there is access to privacy to collect the urine (usually at home or in private work settings), and it must be timed to be completed when there is ready access to an open lab for its submission. I have found Sundays work well with a Monday morning drop-off.

Second, the completion of the collection itself requires these following considerations if it is to accurately portray a 24-hour sample. Think of it as starting out with the bladder dry or empty and finishing with the bladder dry or empty. For the sake of discussion, let's say that a 24-hour collection will be dropped off at the lab at 9 A.M. on Monday morning. At 9 A.M. on Sunday morning, you should urinate and it should be discarded (flushed), as that was urine made since you voided at 6 A.M. or so and is outside the 24 hours of interest. Again, we have now started with the bladder dry or empty. Now for the next 24 hours, every void is collected and placed in the specimen container. Many patients prefer to arrive at the lab and provide their last contribution to the 24-hour collection (in our example at 9 A.M., Monday). We have completed the 24-hour collection with the bladder dry, the final specimen representing the urine manufactured in the concluding 2 or 3 hours of the 24 hours of interest. While it may seem silly that I just explained the principles of a 24-hour urine collection, it is frequently a source of delayed or inaccurate treatment if performed incorrectly.

CALCIUM STONES

Let's now refer to our algorithm (flow diagram) which refers to 100 patients who already have passed a calcium stone (See Figure 17-5). Five will have abnormalities in their bloodwork from conditions which put too much calcium in the blood. This means the kidneys will filter more calcium out in the same volume as a normal, non-stone-forming individual, and therefore present too much calcium to stay suspended. These include:

1.) Hyperparathyroidism--overactivity of a gland in the neck next to the thyroid gland that controls how much calcium is absorbed by our intestine and is lost by the kidneys into urine. This is more common in young women.

2.) Vitamin D and C Toxicity--ingestion of too much Vitamin D and C yields calcium stones; So pay attention, all you vitamin freaks!

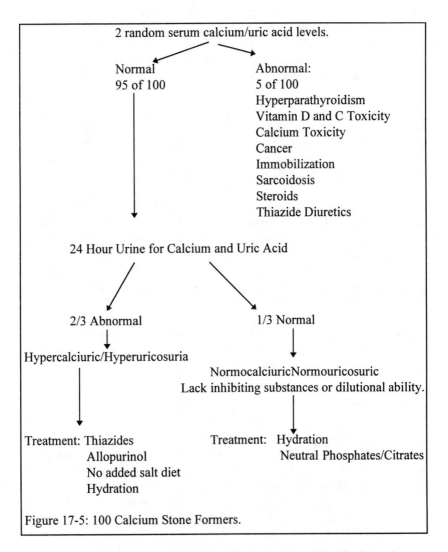

Figure 17-5: 100 Calcium Stone Formers.

3.) Calcium Toxicity--otherwise known as Milk Alkali Syndrome, but involves ingestion of too much calcium, the two most common sources being excessive dairy products or excessive calcium containing antacids.

4.) Cancer--particularly if it has spread to bone and is actively destroying the bone, placing the calcium into the bloodstream.

5.) Immobilization--occasionally as the strength and well-being of the bones are lost from crippling illness, a "demineralization" occurs leading to weakened bones and an overload of calcium into the bloodstream.

6.) Sarcoidosis--a relatively uncommon disease of unknown cause and no true cure frequently has associated elevated calcium and calcium stones.

7.) Steroids--prescribed and illicit can cause bony changes and demineralization.

8.) Thiazide Diuretics--a treatment for blood pressure and interestingly, one of our treatments in the next section for elevations of calcium in the urine have been implicated on occasion for elevations of calcium in the serum.

Each of these conditions requires a different treatment and is beyond the scope of this discussion. As they are conditions outside of a primary genitourinary problem, (that is, the kidney stones actually reflect a symptom of a broader condition), they usually require the involvement of a non-urologist physician as well in their treatment.

Of the remaining 95 calcium stone-formers, two-thirds will have elevations of calcium in their 24-hour urine collection. These form stones because they have too much calcium in their urine to keep suspended, despite maintaining normal levels of calcium in their blood. This occurs either because they absorb too much from their intestinal tract, so called "absorptive" hypercalciurics, or they fail to reabsorb calcium back into the bloodstream which was initially filtered in the first part of the nephron, so called "renal leak" hypercalciura (Refer to Stones Formation, Chapter 17A). Both of these specific subgroups are treated relatively the same, and therefore their separation by further testing is really not necessary unless initial management fails to limit active stone formation.

The treatment of this group entails maintaining a good state of hydration to allow the production of a minimum of 2000 ml. of urine output per day, in males preferably 2500 ml. per day. All stone formers should be particularly attentive to evening fluids as well, drinking enough fluid within the last few hours before bedtime to be awakened at least once if not twice from their sleep to void, insuring that they will be accomplishing adequate dilution.

In addition, there should be the elimination of dietary excess of calcium. The normal American daily diet has 1200 to 1400 milligrams of calcium in it. With approximately 800 mgs. lost in our stool and another 250 mgs. lost in the urine of females and 300 mgs. in male urine, this leaves 100 to 300 mgs. deposited in bone or used for other purposes each day. Supplementing these levels through dietary excess or vitamin supplementation saturates the urine and should be avoided unless under a physician's direction and dictated by other medical conditions, i.e. pregnancy or post-menopausal osteoporosis.

While we're on the subject of dietary excess, a word regarding vitamin C is in order. Vitamin C is metabolized to oxalate and combines to form calcium oxalate stones. Therefore, loading the system increases the oxalate in the urine and increases the likelihood of forming stones, in addition to being a financial waste. Any more than 500 mgs. and certainly more than 1000 mgs. ingested per day is flushed down the toilet.

To monitor the success of a fluid program in maintaining adequate urine output, periodically urine should be collected for 24 hours in the manner discussed earlier for a volume measurement only. This can be done at home. If the volume is considerably less than 2000 to 2500 ml., then more fluids need to be ingested. Stone formers should have their own "jug" in the refrigerator, and it should become reflex to go to the refrigerator for a glass of water to equal (plus some) the amount just voided. Patients who have stone forming tendencies are counseled to increase their fluid ingestion in the latter half of the evening as well, such that their bladder "beckons" them from their sleep at least once per night. During sleep we are relatively dehydrated because we do not have fluids coming on board. This time of sleep would place the patient at risk for the formation of crystals and added stone growth.

Any fluids are good with the exception of dairy products, alcohol (for social conscience reasons), and soft drinks of the "cola" variety as these contain oxalate which combines with calcium to form the most common type of calcium stone. Remember insensible losses, losses through evaporation from skin or moisture in the air we exhale, will dramatically increase during warmer months. Thus, the "stone season" dictates a marked increase in the fluids required to maintain adequate urine output during the warmer months. It is wise to check the 24-hour volume of urine made with changes in seasons or travels to warmer climates to be sure that adequate hydration is accomplised to prevent more stone formation.

In addition to the "behavior modification" techniques, two medications are instituted. One is a thiazide diuretic, which, when teamed with a no-added salt diet, relatively dehydrates the system causing the kidney to resorb calcium from the urine back into the bloodstream. This, in effect, lowers the amount of calcium in the urine and prevents what's left from crystallizing out. The second medication is one commonly used in the treatment of gout. Allopurinol lowers the amount of uric acid in our urine (See more later on Uric Acid Stones). Frequently, uric acid is elevated along with calcium and the two together form stones much more quickly than either alone (synergism).

The final one-third of our 100 calcium stone-formers have neither abnormalities in the blood nor in the urine. These are thought to form stones either on the basis of not diluting their urine enough because of low volume, or they lack inhibiting substances which are chemicals our body manufactures in order to increase the amount of calcium which can be suspended in a given volume of urine. A majority of patients in this group can be treated by hydration alone. Some will require medications which increase solubility, i.e. orthophosphates and citrates.

The above evaluation and treatments will adequately diagnose and treat better than 80% of calcium stone formers. The remaining 15 to 20% may require additional evaluation and specialized treatments in order to prevent recurrence, and truly are beyond the scope of this book. For example, exceedingly rare is the inherited disorder of primary hyperoxaluria rendering early and aggressive stone formation and developing renal failure and death generally by 40 years of age.

WHAT IF I DO NOTHING?

What is the overall likelihood of forming additional kidney stones in the untreated patient? If you take 100 individuals with their first stone and assuming that when they present they have only one stone, their likelihood of passing a second is approximately 70% within 7 years if they are between the ages of 20 and 45 years. Therefore, if we evaluated all 100 initially, we would be putting 30% unnecessarily through the time and expense of a metabolic evaluation. With a second stone, the likelihood of passing a third if untreated is nearly 100%. Therefore, these are the indications for pursuing a metabolic evaluation:

1.) A second stone or a previous history suspicious for stone passage, even though perhaps the stone was not retrieved.

2.) Multiple stones upon initial presentation.

3.) An initial stone which requires surgical intervention In other words, there's worry that this stone grew quickly and sizably because of a very active metabolic process.

4.) Family history of stone disease.

5.) Medical illnesses or medications which would predispose to stone disease.

6.) Any infection stone (See Struvite Stones later in this chapter.) These two processes (metabolic and infectious) can work together to yield extraordinarily rapid stone growth. 20% of patients with infection stones also have a metabolic problem.

7.) Single kidney in an initial stone former.

The age factor tempers the indication for a full metabolic evaluation as the incidence dramatically declines in the sixth decade and beyond.

Monitoring patients currently under treatment involves careful checking of the medical history to elicit suspicion of active stone formation and passage, urinalyses to check for crystals and appropriate urine acidity, and a periodic xray to assess any new stone formation or careful measurement of existing stones to assess any active addition to stone burden. Patients on certain medications require periodic bloodwork to insure there are no abnormalities resulting from the treatment itself, i.e. thiazide diuretics can cause the potassium level in our bloodstream to decline, making us more at risk for irregular heart rhythms. Repeat 24-hour urine collections are performed after the behavior modifications and medication treatments are in place to assess the control of the metabolic abnormality. If a patient has passed only one stone and is without any risk factors for recurrence, the patient will be followed for 5 to 7 years with a single xray performed annually. If everything goes well, the patient will be released at that time. Any patients in the high risk group, i.e. defined metabolic derangements or associated medical conditions which predispose to stone formation, are basically at risk for life.

URIC ACID STONES

These account for approximately 10 to 15% of patients. They are associated in 20 to 40% of patients with gout or gout conditions. These stones are radiolucent, meaning they are not discernible on xray. Frequently, a stone may be outlined by contrast, yielding a "filling defect" to allow the diagnosis.

Patients with uric acid stones, in addition to excreting excessive amounts of uric acid in the urine (greater than 750 mgs. per 24 hours in women and 800 mgs. per 24 hours in men), almost invariably have acidic urine (low pH). Again, the lower the pH, the more acidic the urine. Treatment of these patients centers around increasing urine volume, lessening the amount of uric acid in the urine, and raising the urine pH (making it more alkaline)--all of which increase the solubility of uric acid.

Lowering the body's production of uric acid by dietary adjustments means lessening the protein load, namely elimination of dietary excess of red meats. As discussed earlier, allopurinol decreases the production of uric acid, and alkalinization can be achieved through the use of sodium bicarbonate or potassium citrate. A urinary pH of 6 or greater will adequately prevent the crystallization of uric acid and the formation of stones.

Occasionally patients with an increased metabolism, i.e. patients undergoing chemotherapy or patients post-operative from any major surgery, will present with a uric acid calculus.

INFECTION (STRUVITE) STONES

This process can ravage a normal kidney in very short order. The combination of infection and potential obstruction from a stone lodged in a position to prevent drainage of a kidney can make a patient become very sick, very fast (See Chapter 24, Infections of the Urinary Tract). It is a vicious cycle of stone predisposing to infection and infection predisposing to stones. Very alkaline urine (high pH) is the rule here. In fact, any patient with a urine pH of 7.5 or greater should have a urine culture performed to see if they have an infection with one of the notorious organisms which form these stones. If the culture is positive for infection, at least a plain xray of the kidneys is advisable to rule-out the presence of a silent struvite stone. These stones are composed of magnesium ammonium phosphate and as such will have characteristically a very pungent urine. Stones may be single, multiple, or huge in the configuration of the lining of the kidney occupying part or all of this space, like a plaster model (staghorn calculi).

Treatment principles center around the complete removal of all stone material and aggressive antibiotic therapy once achieved for prolonged periods of time, perhaps life. These patients also warrant a metabolic evaluation to ensure no contribution from metabolic derangement as well.

While not exclusive to this group, a significant percentage of these represent patients with some form of impaired or altered urinary drainage, i.e. the multiple sclerosis patient with impaired bladder emptying or the patient whose urine drains into a bag from a stoma created at the time his bladder was removed for cancer.

CYSTINE STONES

This is an inherited disorder afflicting 1 in 20,000 individuals in the general population in which 4 amino acids, which are the building blocks of all proteins in our body, are excreted to excess into the urine. Of these, cystine is the least able to stay suspended. These stones typically begin to form in the second and third decades. They have a characteristic hexagonal crystal under the microscope, and a "ground glass" appearance on xray. A 24-hour urine for cystine renders the diagnosis. Treatment can be brutal. These patients require very strict dietary limitations, aggressive hydration and alkalinization of the urine, and if necessary the use of some very toxic medication, i.e. D-penicillamine or MPG

SUMMARY

While archeologic evidence demonstrates the earliest of "physicians" curiosity with stone disease, the affliction itself has changed little over the thousands of years since the time of those most astute diagnosticians, utilizing the clinical skills with little to no support by testing and only the crudest of procedures for treatment. Our current medical and surgical management has allowed more accuracy in the diagnosis of urolithiasis, less invasive treatment for stones, as well as lessening recurrence through better preventative medicine. As with most ailments, patient compliance to treatment remains key to successful management of a disease which is 70 to 80% preventable.

CHAPTER 18

KIDNEY TRANSPLANTATION AND DIALYSIS

Treatment for end-stage kidney disease.

Many diseases affect the ability of the kidneys to serve as adequate filters of toxins, normal products of our bodies' metabolism, and excess fluids our bodies' carry. The failure to provide this service may be acute (that is, all of a sudden) or it may be chronic and progressive. The end point at which the combined function of both kidneys can no longer provide adequate filtering to sustain the patient is called End-Stage Renal Disease (ESRD). Amazingly, although dependent upon the specific disease process, approximately 10% of normal kidney function is adequate to keep a patient off of dialysis. Said another way, the kidneys provide us with approximately 90% filtering reserve. At or shortly before this point, if it can be anticipated, dialysis and/or transplant, is planned and implemented.

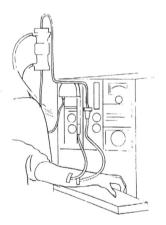

Figure 18-1: Hemodialysis performed upon blood through
mechanical assistance.

Dialysis is the filtration process provided through the mechanical assistance of a machine or through solutions infused into the belly cavity. The former is the more traditional route (called hemodialysis, hemo:blood, + dialysis:filtering) and consists of an access to the patient's circulatory system, generally through a "shunt" which has been surgically created in the patient's arm (See Figure 18-1). The access requires needle puncture. The blood then is pumped through a machine in which the impurities are filtered out, and the blood is returned to the patient's circulation. This is usually supervised by a nephrologist, an internal medicine physician who specialize in disorders of the kidney. By looking at the patient's chemistry studies and weight performed before each dialysis, the nephrologist can fine-tune the dialysis for the needs of the patient that day. Generally, patients are dialyzed one to three times per week, depending upon their own residual kidney function and other medical problems, and each takes approximately one to three hours.

Another less commonly known form of dialysis is called peritoneal dialysis. In this form, an access is placed into the belly cavity by using a small plastic

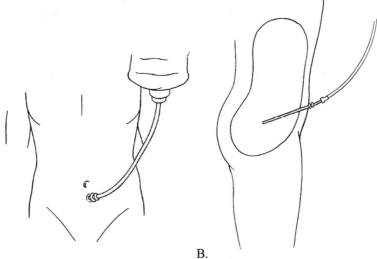

A.   B.

Figure 18-2: Peritoneal dialysis performed through the abdominal
cavity.

access port which has been surgically placed and can be used repeatedly. This allows specially prepared solutions, again tailored to the needs of the patient at that time, to be infused into the belly cavity. The fluids are allowed to reside there for several hours and then are drained, taking with them the toxins, metabolites, and excess fluids.

Kidney transplantation is the placement of a kidney into the body for functional use as the primary organ of filtration. There are certain conditions wherein the patient's own kidney is taken out, operated upon, and replaced (auto-transplantation), however kidney transplantation is generally thought of as placement of either a living donor's kidney or a cadaver donor's kidney, i.e. a brain-dead victim of an accident, into the patient with end-stage kidney disease. The ESRD patient need not have his or her own innate kidneys removed prior to transplantation; although for certain conditions, i.e. uncontrollable hypertension, chronic pyelonephritis (kidney infection), or huge cystic kidneys, this may be necessary.

The transplanted kidney is placed in a pocket created in the lower abdomen and is attached to the patient's own blood supply through an artery and vein and to the patient's bladder by use of the ureter which drains the urine from the transplanted kidney (See Figure 18-3).

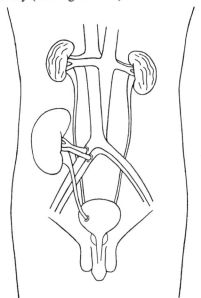

Figure 18-3: The positioning of the transplanted kidney.

Since the mid 1950's when the first human transplant was performed, advances have continued to improve the success and to expand the eligibility for transplantation. The success rates of transplants has continued to improve and nearly 10,000 kidney transplants were performed in the U.S. in 1990. This now represents a very sophisticated sub-specialty involving urologists, general surgeons, and nephrologists. The successful functioning of a kidney 1 year after transplant now approaches 80 to 85%, and patient survival (which in the past had been considerable lower because of immune suppression) is greater than 95%.

The eligibility "requirements" for kidney transplantation include the following:

1.) under age 70;
2.) permanent, irreversible renal failure;
3.) a reasonably normal functioning bladder;
4.) "relatively" free of serious other problems related to kidney failure, i.e. blood vessel, heart, or neurologic problems;
5.) individual consideration if younger than 1 year or older than 70.

The recipient evaluation includes a complete medical history and physical exam, diagnostic/ laboratory tests, and important infection testing, including hepatitis screening, HIV testing, VDRL test (a screen for syphilis), and CMV titers (a rare virus) as the patient will be immunosuppressed for transplantation to reduce rejection. If other potential problems exist, they are evaluated early in the process, i.e. gastrointestinal studies if there's concern for an ulcer or cardiac testing if there's concern for heart disease. Specific urologic testing to assure normal functioning of the urinary tract other than the kidneys may be ordered, i.e. cystoscopy (look in the bladder), urodynamics (study of the tone of the bladder), and voiding cysoturethrogram (xray study to assure no obstruction to urine flow and to assure no backup to the kidneys of urine during voiding, called reflux). At this point if a potential donor(s) is(are) available, histocompatibility testing is performed.

To a significant extent, the success or failure of transplant is not limited to the surgical ability to "hook up" another's kidney in the ESRD patient. Rather it is dependent upon the accuracy in determining the compatibility between the donor's tissues and those of the patient and in managing or limiting the incompatibilities between the two. Pre-transplant blood testing now includes Histocompatibility Testing which determines the degree of tissue compatibility between the donor and recipient. A perfect match is called a 6 antigen match and obviously points favorably to a successful transplant. Traditional Blood Group Matching (ABO System) is necessary for transplant. Cross Matching is testing for the presence of antibodies (key mediators in an immune response) in the recipient which would react to the donor's tissues, i.e. "pre-sensitized" by pregnancy, transfusion, or even previous transplant. A useful test particularly in the selection of a living, related donor is the Mixed Leukocyte Culture in which white blood cells, the soldiers in the immune battle, of the donor and recipient are mixed in the laboratory and stimulated to react.

The patient without a potential donor must wait for a kidney from a a cadaver donor and is placed in the United Network for Organ Sharing (UNOS) system which assigns a point system based upon specific criteria, i.e. histocompatibility match, waiting time, medical urgency, and age to name a few.

Donor evaluation includes those items basic to safe surgery for the donor and successful recipient transplantation, but it is also very important to have psychologic and sociologic assistance with this very stressful dynamic of a loved one with a need for transplantation. The risks and complications of transplant surgery must be clearly understood and undertaken without pressure to provide the kidney. The decision not to donate must not be questioned and in some cases needs to be protected of its confidentiality behind a medical reason. No one morally or ethically can be "forced" to donate an organ.

Organ availability, clearly, limits kidney transplant. In 1990 approximately 8,600 cadaver kidneys, harvested from individuals who were brain dead, were transplanted, yet 175,000 ESRD patients remained on dialysis. As of February, 1992, nearly 20,000 individuals awaited transplant in the U.S. Better awareness in the public sector would enable this decision to be made by the donor well in advance of his/her catastrophic automobile accident, for example, and would free the physicians, nurses, and the transplant team from the extremely difficult task of approaching a family at their time of grief to ask for such a donation. Currently, many kidneys and other organs are not salvaged for this very reason. If, however, the individual had made a conscious decision to do this if ever the need arose, the family's burden, as well as that of the transplant team, would be lifted. One solution is better awareness, perhaps as a mailing in advance prior to the renewal of the driver's license.

Cadaver donor selection begins with an assessment of the overall suitability with regards to nature of the injuries, other medical illnesses and history, and the meeting of very stringent criteria for brain death, including the need for 2 physicians to pronounce the patient one of whom must be a neurologist or neurosurgeon and neither of whom can be part of the transplant team. If these criteria have not been met, the potential donor is managed to optimize his or her survival even if such treatment may in fact lessen the likelihood, or eliminate entirely, the patient as a suitable donor. Organ procurement is the surgical procedure in which all suitable tissues and organs are harvested to be used in transplant. Once harvested the compatibility testing is initiated, and the results are promptly computer analyzed to review any potential local recipients who might be a suitable match. If none is found, the availability of the organ(s) are made national through the UNOS system, and the organs are express-shipped to the transplant institution servicing the best candidate. As this system has developed, so have the techniques of organ preservation and storage.

Incredible advances have been made in this medical discipline and place us at the edge of uniformly offering preservation of life through transplantation. Paradoxically, this comes at a time in history when very difficult legislative decisions will affect the management decisions which have been made in the past through a strictly medical thought process. As influences come from outside the doctor-patient relationship, we will continue as a society to painfully, yet necessarily, reshape and reformulate our moral and ethical decision making process in all aspects of medical care, but particularly in the transplantation arena.

For more information write or call: The National Kidney Foundation, 30 East 33rd Street, 11th Floor, New York, New York, 10016; (800) 622-9010, or National Kidney and Urologic Diseases Information Clearinghouse (NKUDIC), Box NKUDIC, Bethesda, MD., 20892; (301) 468-6345.

CHAPTER 19

SCROTAL CONCERNS

Masses of the male genitals.

A brief discussion of the development of the external genitalia will assist not only in the understanding of this chapter, but it will also lead to a better comprehension of the parallel structures between the female and the male anatomy.

The development in the womb is set up to automatically produce a female (XX). The genetic coding provided in the sex chromosomes determining a male (XY) allows the development of the testicles. The testicles form originally in an area to each side near the kidneys. By seven weeks of development this formation process is complete. The testicles then exert their influence upon the development of a normal male in three very important ways. First, they follow a path of descent into the scrotum which is only completed within the last 4 to 6 weeks of development. Second, they produce testosterone (the male hormone), which travels via the fetus' bloodstream to the area which will become the genitals. This serves to stimulate these cells to form the structures which will become the penis and scrotum. Third, the testicles manufacture a substance called Mullerian Inhibiting Factor (MIF). This substance prevents those areas destined to become the uterus, fallopian tubes, and top one-third of the vagina from developing. Remember, the

system is automatically set up to form a female unless otherwise directed. In the female's development, there is no direction to form a testicle, and therefore an ovary develops. There is no MIF, and therefore the uterus, tubes, and top one-third of the vagina form; and there is no testosterone, so the external structures and lower two-thirds of the vagina develop into a normal female. Refer to the analogous structures between the male and female (See Figure 19-1).

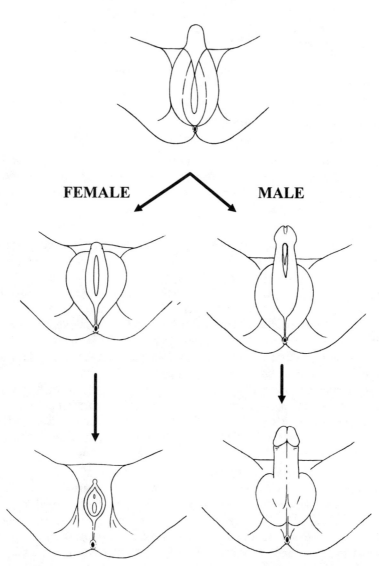

FEMALE

MALE

Figure 19-1: The analogous structures of the male and female genitalia.

AMBIGUOUS GENITALIA

Occasionally, children are born with genitalia which are somewhere in between a male and female. This can be a tremendous source of concern and confusion for the parents. Aberrations in the development may be directly related to some flaw intrinsic to the structures themselves, i.e. the cells destined to be the penis and scrotum did not respond to the stimulation provided by normal testosterone from normal testicles or an error occurred in the manufacturing of hormones by the adrenal glands of the fetus which secondarily affected the genitalia's development, or the aberration may have resulted from some outside source, i.e. an exogenous chemical exposure, including drugs, medications, smoking and alcohol which the mother exposed her fetus to during early pregnancy.

Genetic assignment is not difficult--a scraping of the inside of the infant's cheek to obtain cells for analysis (Buccal Smear) can detect the presence or absence of the Barr Body, or extra X chromosome. Phenotypic assignment, in other words, the sexual assignment which the child will live out in social behavior, is considerably more difficult. If the child is genetically a female, correction of the hormonal imbalance and generally less extensive surgery will render a very good, functioning result. With males genetically, the decision to maintain male sexual assignment is generally based upon if the penis is thought to be of adequate size to be functional. If not, then a female sexual assignment will be better for the infant, and surgical correction can be performed including the removal of the testicles. While the child will obviously be an infertile female, she will be able to function well socially, psychologically, and sexually as a female. Obviously necessary is complete psychologic counseling for the parents to help in the acceptance of the decision and counseling for the child, especially later in life, to understand her infertility due to absence of a uterus and ovaries.

HYPOSPADIAS

Hypospadias, a disorder specific to the development of the urethra of the penis (tube through which the urine travels) and its failure to develop out to the tip of the penis, is discussed separately in Chapter 4.

CRYPTORCHIDISM (UNDESCENDED TESTICLE)

The testicle descends from its origins near the kidneys, and in doing so takes its blood supply from this area (See Figure 19-2). Blood supply into the testicle (the gonadal artery) and blood draining from the testicle (the gonadal veins) both are serviced near the kidneys. This will be important in a later discussion on a condition called a varicocoele. As well, lymphatic vessels,

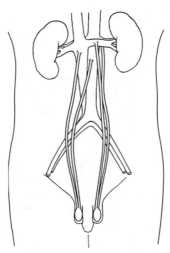

Figure 19-2: The blood supply of the testicle.

which are the filters, drain parallel to the blood vessels and enter into lymph node chains near the kidneys. This will be important in our discussion of cancer of the testicle.

The testicle rests at the top of the inguinal canal (groin) by 3 months of development in the womb. The final descent occurs over 2 to 3 weeks in the last 4 to 6 weeks of pregnancy. Overall, approximately 3.5% of males born have one or both testes undescended. Premature infant males have a much higher incidence because of this late normal last portion of descent with nearly 20% incidence if 2000 grams birth weight and nearly 100% if less than 1000 grams birth weight (3500 grams is a normal birth weight.). Bilateral, or both, testes are undescended in 10% of undescended testicle patients. Another way of subdividing cryptorchidism is that 65% reside in the inguinal canal (groin crease) or below, 15% reside just inside the abdominal wall (internal ring), 15% reside between this ring and the kidney. Only 5% are truly absent. This means that with an absent testicle by examination, we are 95% certain that it is present but not appreciable by inspection or to the touch, and we are obligated to locate it and place it in its correct position.

The most common reason why a testicle does not reside in the scrotum is called a "retractile testicle". As the testicle descends, it takes with it some muscle fibers from each of the 3 layers of muscle of the belly wall. These allow the testicle to be drawn up when the child is cold or scared. Unclothed and cold in the doctor's office then, it's not surprising that, on occasion, it might be difficult to find a testicle by examination of a young boy. Frequently, the parents will relay that both are readily apparent when the child is taking a warm bath. If the testicle can be manually brought into the scrotum, then it will reside there permanently when growth of the testicle and elongation of its cord have occurred.

An easy way to check for a testicle which is not apparent in the scrotum is the following: Place your calm and warm child on his changing table. Place some lotion on your index and middle fingertips. Begin at the bony prominence called the anterior superior iliac spine with the fingers parallel to the groin crease and roughly pointing at the penis. With gentle pressure slide your fingers along pushing anything of a grape-like texture and slightly smaller ahead of your fingertips. If it's low, you will be able to feel the

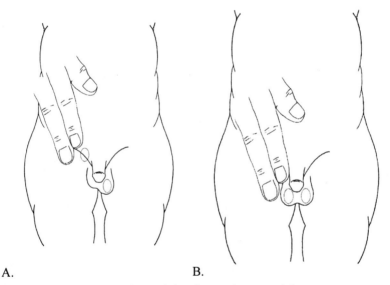

A.   B.

Figure 19-3: Techniqe of examining for an absent testicle.

testicle in the scrotum with your fingertips of the other hand. If it's higher, your fingers will appreciate the bulge but probably will not be able to advance the testicle into the scrotum. Of course, there is no substitute for having your physician confirm this for you. This is just too important of a diagnosis to just assume it is retractile and will descend later.

What is the concern for an undescended testicle? Stated in another way, what are the goals of operating upon a child with cryptorchidism (crypt: mystery, + orchid: testicle)?

First, the testicle must be placed in a position to be examined, by physicians, by parents, and by the patient eventually with self-exam. An undescended testicle is 25 to 50 times more susceptible to the development of testes cancer. and its risk is dependent upon where the testicle is located. The higher the testicle, that is, the less it descended on its own, the higher the risk. Placing it into the scrotum surgically does not diminish this potential, but it does place the testicle into a position for earlier detection. The risk is so low that it certainly would not require that all boys with undescended testicles have them removed. There is a latency period for the development of cancer, developing usually between the ages of 20 to 45 years. Thus, it is imperative that even the boy who has had successful surgery to place the testicle into the scrotum be taught the principles of good self-exam when old enough to understand, usually around puberty. Thereafter, a good gonadal exam should accompany EVERY physical exam by a physician.

The second reason to place the testicle in the scrotum: to protect future fertility. The testicles' positions in the scrotum keep them approximately 2 degree Centigrade cooler than core body temperature, necessary for optimal sperm production. Cryptorchid testes are approximately core body temperature, and as such, undergo changes which are unmistakable under the microscope by age 3 years. Two rules apply: The longer a testicle is left undescended, the less fertile; and, the higher the testicle, the less fertile. Most urologists agree that the testicle(s) should be brought down by age 2 years. While the best chance for self-descent is within the first 3 to 4 months after birth, 75% of full-term boys with cryptorchid testes and 95% of premature infant boys with cryptorchid testes will self-descend by age 1 year. If not down by age 1 year, it is advisable to proceed with surgical correction, certainly completed by age 2 years. Also, beyond age 2 years and certainly by age 3 years, genital surgery is more psychologically upsetting to the child as the genitals have been strongly incorporated into the child's psyche. Separation from the parents is also less upsetting if the surgery is completed prior to age 2 years.

The third reason to operate upon an undescended testicle: to correct the hernia which frequently accompanies the undescended testicle. A rough formula for the sides affected is "60-25-15", that is, 60% right, 25% left, and 15% both. A brief discussion of another anatomical relationship is important at this juncture. Think of the belly cavity in which the intestines reside as a grocery sack (Figure 19-3).

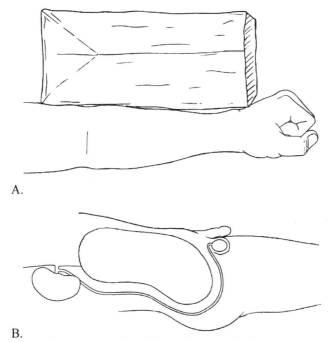

A.

B.

Figure 19-4: The relationship of the testicle and its blood supply with the abdominal cavity.

You have a front wall of the sack and a back wall of the sack, with the groceries themselves analogous to the intestines. Now make a fist and stretch your arm straight ahead of you. Your fist is the testicle and your arm is the "cord", the blood vessels and lymphatics which supply and drain the testicle. Now lay an empty grocery sack, opened but with the bottom end at your wrist, on top of your arm. You now have just constructed the relationship between the testicle, its blood supply, and the abdominal cavity. What happens with normal descent is that the testicle takes a small pinch of this sack with it. The neck of this pinch of tissue usually closes off and it's of no concern. If, however, it remains open and sizable, a hernia is formed in which a protrusion of bowel is allowed to protrude down the groin and into the scrotum. This obviously requires correction to preclude the risk of bowel entrapment in the hernia. If the neck is tight enough to prevent bowel from tracking through but does not seal off completely, fluid from the belly cavity makes its way into the scrotum, billowing it to sizable proportions (See later discussion on Hydrocoele.).

The surgery then is performed in the groin area, like an adult hernia surgery. The testicle is fixed or attached into the scrotum either through the construction of a small pouch in the muscular wall of the scrotum, called a dartos pouch, or by use of a button which is tied to the scrotal skin for several days. Occasionally, and particularly with a high testicle, a two-staged approach (requiring 2 surgeries) spaced over several months may be needed to assure a good intrascrotal positioning. In bilateral (both sides) cases, occasionally a pre-surgical treatment with a chemical called HCG (Human Chorionic Gonadotropin) may assist in gaining some additional length of the cords prior to surgery. This is administered by injections (usually 3 total, given one every other week) and a periodic of observation for several weeks ensues to assess for any additional length gained to make the surgery more likely to succeed. HCG does not seem to be helpful if only one testicle is undescended.

With proper assessment and surgical technique, an overall success rate of testicular salvage and intrascrotal placement should be accomplished with 90% or greater certainty.

HYDROCOELE

The term hydrocoele is applied to a generally painless condition of swelling of a fluid-filled sac in the scrotum. The fluid collects in the 2 layers enveloping the front and sides of the testicle (think of our grocery sack model from above). The fluid separates the layers and engulfs the testicle frequently such that a testicle cannot be clearly identified in the scrotum. In children this process occurs because, as described previously, there is a communicating neck (called a patent processus vaginalis) which allows fluid to track back and forth to the belly cavity.

Astute parents often notice that the testicle and scrotum appear normal when the child first awakens from sleep, when he's been horizontal. But after he's been upright for a few hours of play, the scrotum has enlarged to sizable proportions. This is generally a condition of infants and young children. The testicle is generally descended; and if not detectable by touch, it often can be seen by transillumination, whereby a penlight placed to shine through the scrotum casts a shadow of the testicle within. The surgical timing, principles, and approach are generally those as described for cryptorchidism above. If, however, a hernia is detected, that is, a concern for intestine protruding into the scrotum, then immediate surgery is indicated to prevent incarceration (entrapment with risk of bowel perforation).

Hydrocoeles in adults are slightly different in their cause (etiology) and in their treatment. While similar in that it represents a fluid collection between the layers of the scrotum, in adults there is no track communicating with the belly cavity. The fluid is constantly being produced and reabsorbed in normal adults with the space between the layers being only a potential space. If some process occurs which would prevent the equal and adequate resorption (uptake back into the circulation) of this fluid, the buildup would occur and an apparent hydrocoele forms. This occurs on occasion after scrotal trauma, infection of the testicle, on an idiopathic (no discernible cause) basis, and occasionally with tumor of the testicle.

Frequently, if the testicle cannot be examined reliably and in its entirety, the urologist may order an ultrasound study of the scrotal contents to make sure there is no tumor before exploration. The surgery for an uncomplicated, simple adult hydrocoele is performed through the scrotum, as there is no neck to the abdominal cavity to address unless a hernia is also present. The layers are opened, the fluid drained, and the layers are sewn in such a way to prevent reaccumulation. To demonstrate the surgical principles, lay the grocery sack back on your fist and arm, and now take a scissors and cut the front wall to the sac down the middle and across the bottom (See Figure 19-5). Now fold the edges around to the back side of your fist and arm, in effect having turned the sack inside out. Now, with your third hand or with the help of an assistant, tape the edges to hold that configuration. You have just simulated a "Bottle Technique Hydrocoelectomy". The fluid continues to be manufactured, but will be resorbed by the other layers of the scrotal wall when the testicle and associated structures are replaced into the scrotum, and the space which served as the reservoir to make the scrotum appear swollen has been eliminated.

If there are other complicating features, i.e. an associated hernia or a concern for malignancy (See Chapter 21, Male Self-Exam and Testes Cancer), then an approach through a groin or inguinal incision will be planned by the surgeon, much like with infants and small children. Properly performed

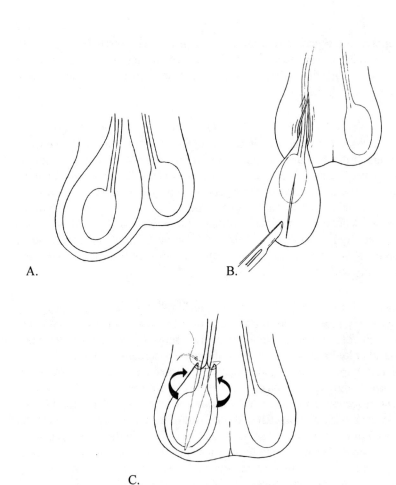

A.

B.

C.

Figure 19-5: The Bottle Hydrocoelectomy.

hydrocoele surgery can be expected to be uniformly successful, completed comfortably in the outpatient setting (particularly with use of local anesthetics in the tissues administered during surgery and expected to alleviate post-operative pain during the first 6 to 8 hours), and with low risk for bleeding or scrotal loss.

There is a period of several days of limited activity, i.e. no straddle activity, but the post-operative disability can be expected to be very limited.

HERNIA

In children, hernias and hydrocoeles are very similar, as described above, with the hernia being a sizeable hydrocoele in as much as the communication to the belly cavity is sizeable enough to allow bowel to bulge into the scrotum. Generally the muscular architecture of the belly wall is good, unlike adults. A hernia in an adult begins then with a laxity of the muscles of the belly wall which "contain" the belly cavity. If this integrity is lost, then the abdominal cavity will "pouch out" at the point of weakness. This is akin to taking a partially blown up balloon and squeezing it between your hands. Wherever it's not contained, it will puff out. Hernia repairs of many types, performed in a classic incision or through the laparoscope, performed with or without the use of some foreign material called mesh, all are directed at shoring up the weakness as a means to control size and pain and to prevent the entrapment of bowel within the hernia sac.

VARICOCOELE

A varicocoele is best described as a "bag of worms" within the scrotum. It is made up of a collection of dilated veins surrounding the testicle which takes the texure of a bag of worms. Recall that blood returning from the testicle must travel to nearly the level of the kidneys before entering into the large vessels which return the blood directly to the heart. In the upright position then, there is a sizable hydrostatic head of pressure that must be overcome in order to cover this distance. This is accomplished through the use of valves which function just like the locks of the Panama Canal (See Figure 19-4). As

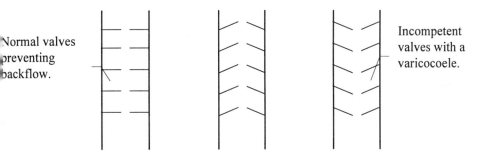

Normal valves preventing backflow.

Incompetent valves with a varicocoele.

Figure 19-6: The flow of blood through the valves of the testicular veins.

The heart pumps (systole), it pushes the blood through theses valves. With the pause and rest (diastole) following each beat, the blood under the influence of gravity settles to its lowest point, only to be pushed further up

175

with the next beat. If these valves are weak or incompetent, like varicose veins of the legs, the blood settles to its lowest point with collection in the veins around the testicle rendering this appearance and texture of a "bag of worms" within the scrotum.

One can check for the presence of a varicocoele by gently placing the fingertips slight above the testicle while standing upright. In this position then grunt and hold it, as if grunting to lift a heavy object. If scrotum fills more and has the characteristic texture described above, then the diagnosis is a varicocoele.

What's the concern with this condition? It must be understood that this is very common--found in nearly 15% of all male recruits entering the military. Therefore, not all boys or men with this condition will require a surgical correction. However, there are fairly clear-cut indications to proceed with surgery to correct a varicocoele.

In the pediatric age group, a varicocoele should be corrected if:

      1.) there is an appreciable size difference in the testicles themselves (with the involved side expected to be smaller);

      2.) as the boy proceeds through puberty, the testicle seems to lag in its expected increase in volume;

      3.) the size is massive and concerning for catastrophic bleeding should trauma occur; and finally,

      4.) pain is persistent and limiting physical activities, then surgery is indicated.

With adults the indications are similar, except that we would not expect to see an appreciable increase in testicular volume with correction of the adult varicocoele. More importantly, varicocoele is the second most surgically correctable cause of male infertility (Vasectomy ranks number one(!)--correctable by a reversal called vasovasostomy). This will be discussed more in Chapter 23, Male Infertility, but, in essence, multiple theories exist for this relationship with the most plausible being that there is a lessening of the normal temperature gradient which exists between the testicle and core body temperature. Spermatogenesis, or sperm production, is impaired by virtue of the warming of the testicle due to the pooled blood surrounding the testicle within the varicocoele.

Surgery can be performed in either the traditional manner through an incision in the groin like a hernia incision or through the laparoscope. Whatever means are used, the goal of the surgery is to ligate or tie off the veins as they traverse from the body wall up to the kidney area. The many veins form a plexus, or tangled network, in the scrotum, but they combine into a few veins as they are followed upward. It is at this point that the surgery is optimally performed, eliminating the back-pressure or hydrostatic distention previously described thus allowing the veins to involute, or shrink back, over time to a relatively normal size. The blood does have alternative pathways to drain into the general circulation through the blood vessels of the pelvis which do not have this problem of hydrostatic pressure contributing to the problem. Performed through the traditional incision approach, the disability for the patient is approximately equal to that of a hernia surgery; performed laparoscopically, the time of disability is considerably less, but the overall cost of the procedure and risk of recurrence or failure may be higher.

Two additional brief considerations are important. Varicocoeles can be bilateral, that is, on both sides. This is particularly important in the infertile patient as both would require surgical correction if one is expected to improve fertility. The other consideration is the "new" varicocoele, that is, the varicocoele which has not been present previously. Occasionally a large tumor pushing on the veins and preventing their optimal drainage will cause a varicocoele. Kidney cancers, particularly on the left side as the left testicular veins generally empty into the veins draining the left kidney, will on occasion present in this way. Varicocoeles caused in this manner generally will not "go down" the way normal varicocoeles do when the patient lies flat. Any new varicocoele should be brought immediately to your physician's attention.

SPERMATOCOELES

As the name implies, these are sperm-filled cysts which present as lumps in the scrotum. They are discovered by conscientious self-exam, by accident either by the patient or his sexual partner, or in examination seeking a source for scrotal tenderness. In and of themselves they are usually harmless, occasionally causing some discomfort, particularly if they are struck or compressed, i.e. in crossing one's legs, entrapping the scrotum. They seldom reach significant size, usually smaller than a pea but may occasionally be as large as a grape. I have operated upon one which was grapefruit-sized and completely engulfed the penis.

The biggest concern with spermatocoeles is assuring that they are not testicular tumors. On exam, a spermatocoele should be attached to the epididymis--the fingered-sized fleshy structure which curls from on top of the testicle around behind it and to the lower aspect of the testicle. (See Chapter 21, Male Self-Exam and Testes Cancer.) The lump cannot be clearly separated from the testicle, then it warrants further investigation to rule-out the possibility of testicular cancer. The next step then would be an ultrasound of the scrotum, with spermatocoeles appearing as hollow, with fluid-filled centers and no internal architecture. The testicular architecture one would expect to be normal. With testicular cancer, the epididymis would be expected to be normal but the architecture of the testicle would be aberrant. Obviously, with the potential diagnosis of testes cancer, any lump in the scrotum, regardless of its location or texture, should be brought to a physician's immediate attention for an accurate diagnosis and prompt treatment.

While the exact cause of a spermatocoele is not definitively known, most feel it is a weakness in the wall of the epididymis, which then ruptures, allowing the development of a cyst of sperm which connects with the epididymis through its narrow neck (See Figure 19-5). The rupture may have initially

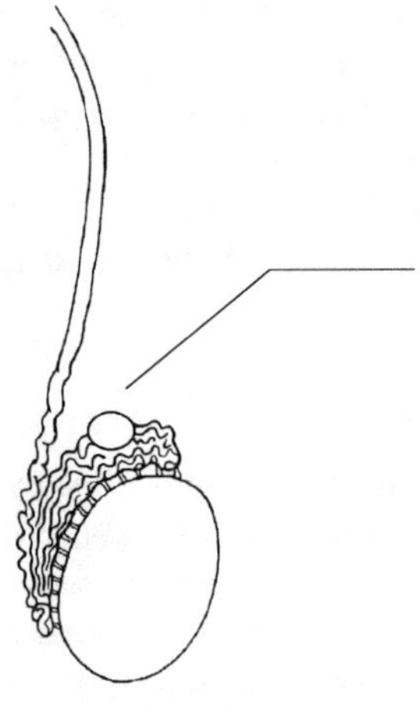

The spermatocoele in the coiled epididymis.

Figure 19-7: A spermatocoele.

occurred unnoticed in the context of seemingly incidental trauma, even sustained during youth. Recall that the epididymis is a coiled single tube which, when stretched out, is more than 18 feet long. The spermatocoele will be positioned next to that part of the epididymis where it formed.

The surgery is designed to remove the lump intact and tie off the neck without disrupting the flow of sperm through the epididymis. Performed through a scrotal approach, unless tumor cannot be ruled out with certainty, it is uniformly successful and performed in an outpatient setting with a minimal amount of post-operative disability. Again, the surgical indications include pain which prevents normal activities, size which prevents reliable examination of the testicle, or exploration to rule out tumor (performed through a hernia-type incision).

LUMPS 'N' BUMPS

Several skin conditions frequently present with scrotal masses which are intrinsic to the scrotal skin or wall of the scrotum. Sebaceous cysts are generally painless masses which are the result of plugged sweat glands which frequently accompany hair follicles. The sebum continues to be secreted by the gland and eventually develops into a noticeable lump which spontaneously ruptures or is brought to the attention of a physician. Generally they are best treated by total excision which can usually be performed with local anesthesia.

Caruncles and furuncles are single or collections of abscess(es), again of the skin, and usually of the sweat gland or hair follicle. These generally are painful and evolve into a mature abscess which will spontaneously rupture or may require surgical drainage. These can be extremely dangerous because certain types of bacteria can spread infection quickly. Without prompt and aggressive drainage and debridement (cutting away of infected and dead tissues), there can be widespread involvement of the genitalia with extension onto the belly wall. These require prompt physician evaluation, particularly if the patient has any other medical conditions which would compromise the ability to combat infection, i.e. diabetes mellitus, poor nutrition, poor hygiene, and cancer.

CHAPTER 20

THE ACUTE SCROTUM

Sudden pain in the male genitals.

One of the most concerning evaluations to perform as a physician is the diagnosis of the young male patient with an acutely painful scrotum. The anxiety runs high for the young patient and the patient's parents, and for the physician the possibility of a missed diagnosis and loss of the testicle places a premium upon a correct diagnosis in a minimum amount of time. Epididiymorchitis (an acutely inflamed testicle caused by infection) or testicular torsion (an acute twisting of the testicle's cord providing its blood supply) are the two most likely diagnoses for this condition.

TESTICULAR TORSION

A sudden twisting of the testicle upon its blood supply will result in an acutely painful testicle. Recall that the testicle hangs in the scrotum like a yo-yo on a string. If the yo-yo twists, the string tightens. In the spermatic cord (the thickened structure felt above the testicle in the upper scrotum) are:

     1.) the blood vessels into and out of the testicle;
     2.) the vas deferens which carries sperm in the adult;
     3.) lymphatic vessels; and
     4.) strands of muscles called the cremasteric muscles which
originate from the abdominal wall muscle layers.

Twisting results in a constriction and closure of the blood vessels into and out of the testicle, much like placing a rubber band around a finger. While individual differences exist regarding ability of the testicle to sustain this insult, the statistics are that 90% of testicles twisted (torsed) less than 6 hours will survive unharmed; between 6 and 12 hours, approximately 50% will survive; and, at greater than 12 hours of torsion, less than 10% will survive. Time is of the essence in order to salvage the testicle, yet we do not want to unnecessarily subject the patient to a surgery if the diagnosis can be ruled out by other means.

Two classic scenarios exist for presentation: first, the young boy either shortly before and while undergoing puberty is awakened from his sleep with an intensely painful testicle; second, the boy or young man experiences excruciating scrotal pain which is sustained after what otherwise would be thought of as seemingly incidental trauma, i.e. upon completion of a bumpy bicycle ride. Pubertal changes are associated with a tremendous increase in the volume of the testicle which may, for a period of time, lack total fixation within the scrotum. Therefore, the possibility exists for twisting to occur until the testicle adequately fixes its position in the scrotum. In four series of patients constituting over 375 cases of "acute scrotum" as the initial diagnosis, the diagnosis was overwhelmingly testicular torsion. For children less than 6 years it was an uncommon clinical condition. Within the age group of 6 to 12 years, half had torsed testicles. In the age group of 13 to 18 years, 75% had torsion. In the 19 to 24 year age group, less than 25% had torsion (The remainder had epididymitis).

In the immediate time of the painful event, the scrotum may look entirely normal. There will not be any apparent redness or swelling for several hours. Occasionally, a slight elevation of the involved testicle or a "horizontal lie" may be noticeable to inspection, but these are not highly accurate in diagnosing and certainly should not delay going to the hospital. With several hours of delay, the scrotum will become more inflamed in its appearance with swelling, redness, and pain all readily noticeable.

In the emergency room, the physician will attempt to exam the scrotum for the alignment of the scrotal contents and to attempt to isolate the location of the pain. Admittedly, even for an experienced urologist, this is a difficult exam. If there is concern for the time interval since the onset of pain-- especially as it approaches 6 hours, immediate surgery to untwist the testicle for salvage may be necessary. If there is the luxury of time, then an assessment of blood flow into the testicle can be performed either through a Testicular Scan, in which a small radioactive injection is given (the total dose of radiation the patient sustains is less than one simple chest xray) and an imaging of the testicle is performed. If there is no flow confirming the diagnosis of torsion, it will show up as a cold spot. If its hot, we have confirmed blood flow into the testicle and we are dealing with either an epididymorchitis (See below) or possibly a testicle which has just de-torsed, i.e. like the redness and warmth in your finger after taking the rubber band off. Alternatively, an ultrasound can be performed with a special attachment which can show blood flow into and out of the testicle, visually yielding our diagnosis.

Surgical exploration is performed under general anesthesia. Usually a midline scrotal incision is made through the middle crease called the raphe. The involved side is entered through this incision first, and the testicle is assessed. It is de-torsed and then fixed in the scrotum with sutures to fix it inside the scrotum in a position where it will not twist again. The uninvolved side is fixed at the same time to assure that it will not subsequently torse. Occasionally, the testicle is removed because it has obviously not survived and may pose problems for possible immediate infection and future fertility if left in place. This latter phenomenon occurs because the testicle is an immunological privileged site, that is, our immune system is normally not allowed to "see" the germ cells of the testicle. As a result of the injury, this may not be the case. If left in place, the dead testicle may serve to gear up our immune system against our own sperm, and they may not be as hearty. There is not much debate when it comes to an obviously dead testicle. The debate continues to be discussed regarding the "questionable" testicle, although most would attempt to spare the testicle, arguing that we're dealing with an immediate organ salvage versus only the possibility of future fertility problems.

The recovery time is amazingly short. These boys are frequently discharged within 24 hours and bounce back very quickly. Periodic check of the testicle will provide the assessment necessary regarding its viability. If it "withers on the vine" it will shrink and become only a small knot in the scrotum. If this occurs or if it requires removal at the time of the exploration, there will be ample production of male hormone and sperm by the solitary testicle remaining, provided it is cared for well. Any future concerns should be brought immediately to the attention of a physician as loss of the solitary testicle would result in infertility and subject the boy to monthly injections of testosterone (male hormone) for life. Occasionally, certain activities may be necessarily curtailed, i.e dirt biking or other more traumatic straddle activity.

EPIDIDYMORCHITIS

This group constitutes the other large percentage of patients with an acute scrotum. As deduced from the discussion above, these patients tend to be a bit older, generally 18 and older. In this group the diagnosis was overwhelmingly epididymitis, accounting for better than 80% of the more than 375 patients previously described. Generally, these patients have an associated infection complaint, i.e. symptoms of prostatitis or urethritis (See Prostatitis, Chapter 25; and Venereal Disease, Chapter 26) preceded the onset of the scrotal complaint. While the scrotal pain may be sudden in its onset, generally the patient will note several hours to even a few days of increasing discomfort. An inflamed appearing scrotum is the rule, with swelling, pain, and redness.

Here the exam may be easier as the pain is directly localized to the area of the epididymis, lying generally behind the testicle wrapping up over its top and across the bottom (See Figure 21-1). This area becomes swollen and intensely tender, but is clearly separable by exam from the testicle itself and generally can be assessed to be in its normal anatomic position, thus ruling out torsion. If any doubt exists, the above testing can be ordered. The decision may be made, based upon clinical suspicion and a concern over viability if the diagnosis of torsion is delayed, to explore with the finding upon exploration of an epididymorchitis. This situation is parallel to that faced by the general surgeon who occasionally finds a normal appendix upon an exploration for a presumed appendicitis. Fortunately this happens seldom, but the possibility does exist. The complications suffered are minimal (less than 2% have problems), and the greater harm by loss of a testicle in a non-explored torsion goes without saying.

An additional suspicion for epididymorchitis comes from a urinalysis reflecting the associated urinary tract infection. A check of the urine will be normal with torsion as there is no associated infection or inflammation of the urethra to shed white blood cells into the urine. With epididymitis, because it is an ascending infection which originated within the urethra or prostate, theoretically one would expect the urinalysis to be uniformly positive for infection. Unfortunately this association will be noted only approximately 15% of the time.

Treatment with the diagnosis secured is generally based upon age. In the very young patient, the cause is likely viral but most would treat with a penicillin or related antibiotic. In the sexually active young man, the cause is likely Chlamydia and therefore a tetracycline would be the drug of choice. In the gentleman over 45 to 50, the same organisms causing prostate infections (prostatitis), called the Gram Negative bacteria, are associated, and therefore treatment would be directed at that group with sulfa type or quinolones most frequently employed. Again, teamed with antibiotics would be ice packs, elevation by use of a towel roll under the scrotum; and, in the non-pediatric age group, non-steroidal anti-inflammatories would be employed. Recall that occasionally a testes cancer can present in this way with signs of inflammation rather than a painless lump. Therefore, if things don't improve with what should be appropriate treatment, there is the possibility that testes cancer may be present. Therefore, these boys or men must always be re-examined after the acute pain and swelling have resolved to assure to the patient, parents, and physician that the testicle is normal.

TORSION OF THE "APPENDAGES"

Brief mention should be made that there are small, tear-drop sized and shaped structures, generally one from the testicle and one from the epididymis, called the appendages which can twist mimicking the acute scrotal conditions, testicular torsion and epididymitis, which we've described above. While torsion of the appendages do not require exploration in and of themselves, they can occasionally cause a diagnosis error. The highest likelihood for this diagnosis to be a cause of scrotal pain came in the 7 to 12 year age group in those studies previously reviewed.

CHAPTER 21

MALE SELF-EXAMINATION AND TESTICULAR CANCER

Principles of self-examination and cancer of the testicle.

The importance of male self-examination cannot be exaggerated. The role of early detection in affording the best outcome in any malignancy is no more evident than with cancer of the testes (testicle). Cancer of the testicle is the most common solid malignancy in young men between the ages of 15 to 40. While there occur 5 to 6 breast cancers in females for every 1 testes cancer in males, the two are very similar in that self-examination is imperative for early detection. Women have been very receptive to the concept of self-exam. Men on the other hand are less receptive--there seems to be almost a stigma against the notion of a man touching himself.

Approximately 20% of masses in the testicle are detected by the sexual partner. The embarrassment of the spouse or friend finding a lump should not serve as a deterrent to having a physician render an opinion, even if it's just reassurance that everything is OK. We would much rather have 100 patients reassured than to have missed an opportunity to make an early diagnosis in one. Knowing that frequently men present with a mass found in this way should defuse this embarrassment.

There is also the important responsibility of teaching the patient self-examination on the part of the physician. Physical exams performed for athletic participation allow a particularly useful access to healthy young boys and men who otherwise would not have reason to be seen by a physician. It is a fairly simple exam to learn, and is best learned upon yourself after reading this section. So the next time you're due to have a physical exam, review the principles of the exam taught below with your physician to be sure you have them right and to be sure as a starting point that your exam is normal.

When thinking of the anatomy of the testicle take a small ball, like a golf ball or ping-pong ball, and hold it with your index finger (See Figure 21-1). Turn your wrists away from your body. This alignment of your finger and the ball directly corresponds to the tube system draining the testicle (epididymis) and the testicle.

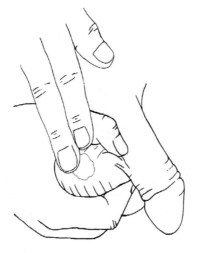

Figure 21-1: The principles of male self-exam.

Self-exam is best accomplished in a relaxed setting, i.e. while lathered up in the shower. The testicle is anchored with one hand, and the index finger of the other hand is used to run gently over the front and side surfaces of the testicle. Both hands are then used to check the back side of the testicle by gently squeezing the soft tubular like structure (the epididymis--your finger in the analogy of holding a small ball with your index finger). Any lumps or areas of tenderness or concern should be brought to the attention of your physician.

All lumps are not malignant (See Scrotal Concerns, Chapter 19). There are may benign conditions which cause a mass in the scrotum. Hernias may cause scrotal enlargement. Hydrocoeles are collections of fluid in the scrotum causing swelling. Varicocoeles are dilated veins, occur more frequently on the left side, and frequently are associated with some tenderness in the scrotum when one is upright for prolonged periods of time. (See Male Infertility, Chapter 23). Lastly, there are cysts in the tube system (epididymis) called spermatocoeles (sperm-filled cysts) which frequently occur and may cause alarm on self-examination. All of these represent benign conditions which far outnumber the tumors to be found. Nonetheless, the exact diagnosis should be made by the physician, and the lump should be assumed to be a tumor until proven otherwise by a physician's opinion.

There are very few identifiable risk factors with testicular malignancy unlike others, i.e. smoking and lung cancer. Two groups come to mind. Any boy who has had surgery for an undescended testicle should have good annual exams including of the testicles and when of an age old enough be taught the principles of self-examination (See Scrotal Concerns, Chapter 19). Even though these operations are accomplished early in life (Urologists are recommending them before age 2 years.), the onset of malignancy is usually much later, into the 20's and 30's. It is imperative that they be counseled as young adults of their increased risk (approximately 40 times more likely when compared to the general population) and the need for self-examination.

The other group are those patients who continue with scrotal complaints (pain and swelling, perhaps mimicking an infection) despite what appears to be appropriate treatment, i.e. antibiotics (See The Acute Scrotum, Chapter 20). Approximately 20% of testes cancer presents with these so called "inflammatory signs" which appear to be a straightforward infections. If there is not a good response to antibiotics, then we evaluate further to rule out the diagnosis of malignancy.

Lastly, in no other tumor has there been as dramatic a turnaround regarding successful treatment as there has been with testicular carcinoma. Fifteen years ago 20% cure rates were the norm--80% succumbed to their disease. We are now affording cures in the range of 70 to 80% cure for all stages of the disease and even 90% cures with limited spread out of the testicle. I would like to report that self-exam has had a serious impact upon these statistics. Unfortunately that just is not the case. The improved cure rate came with better surgical techniques and chemotherapy agents. What this means, however, is that **if men do participate in their health care by self-exam, our cure statistics should improve even more due to earlier detection**.

EVALUATION

With the patient presenting with a scrotal mass, the first evaluation is a physical exam to confirm whether or not the lump is intrinsic to the testicle or can be separated or distinguished from the testicle. Masses which are separable from the testicle are generally benign in nature and fall within one of the diagnoses discussed in Scrotal Concerns, Chapter 19. If however, the mass cannot be distinguished clearly as separate, then the diagnosis is testes cancer until proven otherwise.

Two evaluations promptly follow at that point. First, two blood tests, called tumor markers, are drawn from the arm. Testes cancer, to varying degrees, will manufacture two proteins which are generally detectable in minuscule amounts in the blood of normal males. These two tests are the alpha fetoprotein (AFP) and the beta human chorionic gonadotropin (B-HCG). One or both of these will be abnormal in most testes cancers. The second test, if the physical exam is unclear, is a scrotal ultrasound, a painless test where ultrasonic sound waves are directed at the anatomy in question to show the internal architecture of the scrotal contents. It helps us to delineate whether or not a lump is hollow or solid, and whether it is within, on, or separate entirely from the testicle. The ultrasound, however, does not tell us if the lump is or is not cancer--it is simply a technique of imaging to increase the likelihood of a particular diagnosis.

One additional use of the scrotal ultrasound is in the preoperative evaluation of the patient with a huge hydrocoele or spermatocoele. The entire scrotal contents are obscured by what is presumed to be a benign fluid-filled cyst. To insure that there are no surprises at the time of surgery by the discovery of an unsuspected testes cancer, the ultrasound is sometimes ordered in anticipation of the definitive trans-scrotal (through the scrotum) repair for the non-cancerous condition. This leads us to a discussion of the surgical treatment.

If there is any concern for a potential testes cancer, the surgical approach is through the inguinal area (groin). Recall that the testicle hangs on a cord running through the abdominal wall muscle layers to the origins of its blood supply near each kidney deep within our high back area, actually only slightly below the lowest rib on each side of our back. Approach through the groin allows us, early in the surgical procedure, even before the testicle is handled, to place a tourniquet around this cord, preventing blood flow into the testicle. More importantly, blood flow out of the testicle, which might contain tumor cells and if not contained could spill into the general system depositing elsewhere in the body, is interrupted. Performed in this fashion, if cancer is encountered, the testicle and its cord up to the entry into the belly cavity are removed and is called a radical orchiectomy. If only a biopsy is required and it returns negative for cancer, then the testicle can, after removal of the tourniquet, be placed back into its scrotal position unharmed.

An additional reason for the inguinal area approach to testes cancer has to do with the lymph drainage of the testicle. Recall that the lymphatic system is a drainage system of small channels draining into nodes which filter and kill infection and cancer. The testicle's lymphatic drainage parallels its blood supply, directly up into the deep abdomen surrounding the great vessels to the level of the kidneys. The lymph nodes of the groin area itself (the crease at the junction of the trunk and the leg) are not involved in the drainage of the testicle itself and therefore are spared from cancer contamination. If, however, the scrotum is violated, i.e. an exploration is done through the scrotal wall (trans-scrotal) or a needle is placed through the scrotal wall to obtain fluid for diagnosis, there exists the possibility of tumor spread to these areas. Contamination of the scrotal wall or its draining lymph nodes would require additional surgery or potential complications associated with the cancer's spread to those locations.

An interesting point about testes cancer is that because these are germ cells, (that is, cells which would go on to make sperm), they are totipotential. This means that they may have several different appearances under the microscope and several different biologic behaviors. Therefore, in comparing results or treatments for patients with cancer of the testicle, it is very important that we know exactly the type or combination of types (which frequently occurs) of tumor.

TREATMENT

The likely sites of spread in testes cancer include the lymph nodes of the retroperitoneum (the area behind the abdominal cavity in which the great vessels and kidneys reside). This area (See Figure 21-2) is best examined by the CT (or "cat") Scan. This test involves painless xray which by use of computer technology can construct our internal architecture as if we have been sliced with a sword and turned on end for display. The lungs are depositories as well and are imaged by either the CT Scan or special chest xrays called tomograms.

If there is extensive spread outside the testicle, then chemotherapy is employed. The stalwart treatment is a platinum-based chemotherapy protocol, of which there are several, and which usually involve 2 or 3 different agents. The measure of success is by resolution of the tumor seen on CT Scan and the normalization of the tumor markers. After chemotherapy if a mass remains, then it must be removed to see if it contains any active tumor. One-third will have more of the same tumor or another testes tumor type (remember the totipotential ability) requiring further treatment. The remainder will have a necrotic, benign mass requiring no further treatment. One-third will have a benign, but difficult to treat, tumor called a teratoma.

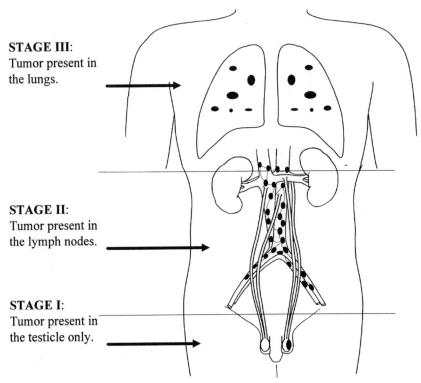

STAGE III:
Tumor present in the lungs.

STAGE II:
Tumor present in the lymph nodes.

STAGE I:
Tumor present in the testicle only.

Figure 21-2: The likely areas of spread for testes cancer.

If all the tests in the metastatic evaluation are negative upon the removal of the testicle by radical orchiectomy, then there is the decision to be made between removal of the lymph nodes through an abdominal surgery to determine if any additional treatment (chemotherapy) is necessary or observation. With observation, monthly tumor markers and chest xrays for the first year (bimonthly for the second year), are performed along with physical examination and periodic CT Scan. If there exists any suggestion of tumor spread, then chemotherapy is employed. Too involved for this introductory discussion, the basic decision here is one of obtaining full treatment in one extended time frame (removal of the testicle followed by surgical removal of the lymph nodes followed by chemotherapy) versus a watch-and-wait posture followed by chemotherapy which may or may not result in additional time of illness and disability over the next 2 to 5 years. The dramatic improvements in survivals and cures afforded by the chemotherapy has allowed the observation choice to be an option, given the patient will subject himself to close follow-up.

One final consideration is a tumor type called a seminoma. It is very sensitive to radiation. Through all the testing and a thorough check of the cancerous testicle, if no other type of testes cancer is found excellent cures are obtained by treatment with radiation. Again, those areas treated are on the route of drainage of the involved testicle.

There's never a convenient time to be ill, especially with cancer. But testes cancer hits at the most productive time of a young man's life--generally between ages 20 to 45, a time for a young family, an aspiring career, and for reaching financial and personal goals. These all can be shattered in an instant with the discovery of testes cancer. Fortunately, while rigorous, the treatments afford a promising outlook for cure, but early detection cannot be understated as critical for a favorable outcome. Encourage your male family members and friends to learn the principles of good self-examination.

CHAPTER 22

VASECTOMY

The procedure for male sterilization.

Vasectomy is the procedure performed upon approximately 500,000 men per year to interrupt the flow of sperm into the ejaculate (that jettisoned upon orgasm or sexual climax). In doing so, the man is rendered infertile (that is, unable to father any additional children). In no way does vasectomy disturb the ability to obtain or sustain erections satisfactory for successful intercourse (potency), nor does it alter any of the sexual satisfaction associated with orgasm. Quite the contrary, many couples relate a more satisfying sexual relationship following sterilization by virtue of eliminating the need for other more cumbersome means of birth control and the risk of pregnancy.

Vasectomy will not alter the appreciable volume, color, or consistency of the ejaculate. The sperm comprise only 2 to 5% by volume of the ejaculate--toss that one out at your next cocktail party! The only way to check for successful sterilization is a microscopic examination of the ejaculate. There is no way to diagnose successful sterilization by just looking at it without microscopic assistance. The test is very easy to do--and it is the ease of checking that makes vasectomy the sterilization procedure of choice. All one must do is obtain a semen check by ejaculating into a cup and submitting it to a laboratory.

The only precautions are that it is best to refrain from sexual activity for a few days before and when the specimen is collected it must be the entire ejaculate. Most couples utilize the "pullout" method to collect the specimen. In doing so, the most likely portion of the specimen to be missed is the first portion. The first portion of the ejaculate, that jettisoned first, has the highest concentration of sperm in the normal unsterilized male. Therefore, in a"post-vasectomy" check, that done after vasectomy, the most likely location for those few stragglers is the first portion. There is no magic time or number of ejaculates after vasectomy that a gentleman becomes sterile. My practice has been to have the gentleman submit a specimen after 20 ejaculates because at that time there is a 92 to 95% certainty of successful sterilization. On occasion there will remain a few sperm seen--but it only takes one of those little guys. If any sperm are seen, the couple is counseled that they are not sterile, and a specimen is rechecked in another 10 to 15 ejaculates or so. If a couple have intercourse seldom, there is nothing magical about 6 weeks or 3 months. For greatest certainty, a specimen must be checked.

Yet in my practice despite being repeatedly and strongly encouraged to complete a semen analysis, nearly 25% fail to do so. A specimen is checked approximately one year from the time that the gentleman is told he's sterile. The failure rate of vasectomy is approximately 5 per 10,000 performed. Those that fail to become permanently sterile do so usually within the first year after the vasectomy. Therefore, if we check a year out from the time of a noted successful sterilization, and the gentleman is still sterile, he is highly likely to remain sterile for the rest of his life unless another factor would enter into the picture, i.e. a severe blow to the scrotum or a bad infection. In this case, once healed or resolved another check of the semen should be performed.

When comparing the risks of performing a vasectomy (male sterilization) versus tubal ligation (female sterilization), the couple must understand that both are done easily and routinely with high success and few failures. Tubal ligation is more invasive involving an entry into the belly cavity to view the fallopian tubes in order to clip them shut. The failure rate of vasectomy is approximately 5 per 10,000 performed, for tubal ligation it is slightly higher at approximately 15 per 10,000 performed. Neither then is likely to fail. But if you consider that vasectomy is less invasive and has a higher success rate, it seems evident why, in the absence of any other complicating medical condition, vasectomy is the preferred means of accomplishing sterilization.

Testing for a successful sterilization is more easily accomplished for vasectomy as described above as opposed to a woman's testing which involves either a pregnancy or an xray test where a liquid contrast is placed in the uterus and tubes to check for patency (openness) of the tubes--both an expensive and uncomfortable test. One final consideration is the reversibility of the procedure. While both are successfully reversed in situations such as a catastrophic loss or desire for additional children or a second family, vasectomy is less invasive and more easily reversed (See Male Infertility, Chapter 23).

We know of no definite long-term untoward (bad) health affects as a result of having a vasectomy. A few years ago there was a much-sensationalized study which proposed to link an accelerated rate of coronary artery disease (hardening of the blood vessels servicing the heart) with vasectomy. This was based upon lab animals simultaneously being experimented upon with a high cholesterol diet. We now know, upon separation of the studies and with the additional work done on cholesterol effects, that the diet, and not the vasectomy was responsible for the heart disease.

More recently attempts have been made to link increased risk of prostate carcinoma in vasectomized men. The American Urological Association has strongly denounced this association with the data now on hand but has not discouraged the continued research to assure that this common procedure has no health risks. Recent epidemiologic studies (studies of large populations of people wherein data is logged into computer data banks and analyzed for any statistically significant associations) suggested a relationship between prostate cancer and vasectomy. This should not be interpreted as a cause and effect. Simply stated, there seemed to be an increased incidence in prostate cancer in men who had been vasectomized for 20 years or longer. The interesting thing to consider here is that most men have their vasectomy in their mid to late 30's. Plus twenty years would make them 50 to 55 years old, the age at which prostate cancer begins to become more prevalent anyway, and at which time all men should begin their prostate cancer screening consisting of an annual rectal exam and a blood test called the PSA (See Prostate Cancer, Chapter 8). The only additional recommendation to come from these more recent studies is for men who have not yet reached the age of 50 and have been vasectomized for greater than 20 years. They should begin their prostate screening earlier, perhaps at age 40 to 45.

With vasectomy there is the development of an immune response (our body's defense system) in which the sperm are recognized as foreign, like a response to an infection. As such 10 to 15% develop anti-sperm antibodies which, in the event that the man desires a return of his fertility, would make the sperm less hardy. Those sperm barraged with this immune response tend neither to be good swimmers nor penetrators of the egg. As well, This immune response goes on even after the plumbing has been "hooked back up", and this phenomenon is directly related to the time through which a man has been vasectomized. Therefore, urologists will ironically counsel a patients in his early twenties not to have a vasectomy in order to protect his future fertility should he have a change of mind, i.e. a change of spouse. Sociologists tell us that a marriage lasting into the thirties has a greater chance of survival than a couple in their twenties. They also tell us that a man who is divorced particularly in the late thirties, or early forties is much less likely to be desirous of a second family than that same gentleman in his twenties or early thirties.

The problem with vasovasostomy (vasectomy reversal) is not one of obtaining sperm in the ejaculate--this can be accomplished in skilled hands better than 70% of the time--but rather is one of obtaining good quality sperm which will be good swimmers and penetrators for successful fertilization. There is no association of vasectomy or its reversal with birth defects. Interestingly a urologist's role with a patient requesting voluntary sterilization can be one of protecting the patient's own compromise of his fertility.

Our neonatologists (pediatrician's specializing in newborn children) and pediatricians tell us that if a child lives for the first year, the likelihood of survival is considerably better than that predicted prior to that age. Therefore, many urologists will inquire and some require that the couple have two children, the younger of which be at least one year of age. In counseling the couple, if they truly would attempt to have another child if they were to suffer the catastrophic loss of one of their children, further deliberation should be allowed before vasectomy is performed. There is another bump in the death rates in children around age 6 to 8 years when they gain more independence and suffer traumatic deaths, i.e. bicycling accidents. No one likes to entertain these thoughts, but they very important considerations before giving up one of our most innate abilities: to procreate.

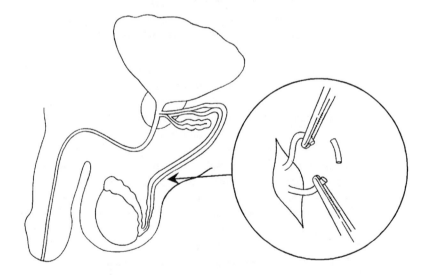

Figure 22-1: Vasectomy.

The performance of a vasectomy is usually quite simple (See Figure 22-1). After sterile preparation of the scrotum (sac containing the testicles), the vas deferens (the tube connecting the epididymis and testicle into the urethra) is gently grasped and brought below the level of the scrotal skin. The remainder of the structures in the spermatic cord (the cord upon which the testicle hangs and also includes blood vessels, lymphatics, and muscle tissue) are separated by palpation or feel so that only the vas deferens will be cut. The skin and vas are then anesthetized (numbed) by injection. A small incision is made, approximately the width of your smallest fingernail. The vas deferens is freed, a small section cut out (maybe one-half inch), and the ends are clipped or tied, all in an attempt to permanently prevent the flow of sperm. The incision is closed with a couple of stitches, most of the time a self-absorbing type not requiring removal. There are many methods for vasectomy, including a recently touted "crush technique", done without incision. In skilled hands, standard vasectomy can be done relatively painlessly and quickly (often less than 20-30 minutes). It is an important decision involving two individuals and potentially a third. Therefore most urologists do not condone these short-cut techniques, i.e. the crush technique or other "no incision techniques, touted for the most-part by non-surgeons.

The instructions given for post-operative care are as varied as the surgeons doing the procedure, so I'll speak only for myself. I have the gentlemans finish their course of doxycycline (an antibiotic) and non-steroidal anti-inflammatory which were begun on the morning of the procedure. This usually takes one week. These were prescribed and initiated before the procedure to minimize the risk of the development of "post-vasectomy epididymo-orchitis," or an inflamed testicle and epididymis, which occurs occasionally after vasectomy (See The Acute Scrotum, Chapter 20). The nonsteroidal antiinflammatory, i.e. ibuprofen, also lessens the pain after the procedure by interrupting the pain cycle before it is initiated. After the vasectomy, the men wear a supporter or support underwear for one week. Also I asked them to refrain from ejaculation for one week. They are asked to stay off their feet as much as possible after the procedure is performed that day. The next day they can be up and around, but I request that they refrain from heavy lifting or physical exercise. They are asked to use an ice-pack for 20 to 30 minutes at a time every 3 to 4 hours for the first 24 hours. They resume normal activities shortly thereafter.

All of these recommendations are an attempt to minimize the risk of post-vasectomy epididymo-orchitis (inflammation of the tube system and testicle) or bleeding. The definition of "macho" is the guy who rides his "Harley®"

home from his vasectomy. I don't care if the guy is "macho", I just want this to go smoothly and to not set up a chronic pain situation if things do not heal optimally. Upon return for a wound check at one week, we reaffirm the need for continued birth control until the semen analysis described above is obtained and shows no sperm.

If the patient continues monthly self-examination, he will note a small knot in the cord above the testicle at the site of the vasectomy which on occasion may become swollen and tender. This is called a sperm granuloma. Sperm granulomas represent the body's immune response to the sperm coming up to the "roadblock", dying, and being digested by our immune system. On occasion sperm granulomas become so tender that surgical excision is required.

Vasectomy allows a reasonable solution to concerns of sterilization. Most of the fear of the procedure is exaggerated because of the sensational stories from "friends". It is almost like the "right of passage" or the initiation into the club. This factor, however, does delay many gentlemans from proceeding, resulting in either no sterilization procedure or the wife's proceeding to tubal ligation. Most of those who proceed with vasectomy find that the anxiety was unnecessary, for most vasectomies are accomplished uneventfully.

CHAPTER 23

MALE INFERTILITY

Male fertility problems.

Fifteen percent of all marriages have a fertility problem, of which approximately 50% are in part or totally referable to a male factor. Any discussion of fertility must be placed in the context of a **couple**, as a super-fertile partner may compensate for a sub-fertile partner, i.e. between 5 and 23% of known fertile males have been found to have low sperm counts and nearly 10% of known fertile men have low sperm motility (the swimming capability of the sperm). A 25% pregnancy rate occurred without treatment in sixteen couples who had unsuccessfully participated in an intrauterine insemination study. This serves as a control to measure successes of any treatment as up to 1 in 4 couples might go on to conceive whatever is done, even nothing.

For the purposes of our text, female infertility will not be discussed here. This problem is treated by gynecologists with a sub-specialty interest in female infertility and female endocrinology (the study and treatment of hormonal abnormalities). Several fine texts and patient informational materials can be obtained through a gynecologist's office or in the medical section of a local bookstore. Any evaluation of female infertility will include at least one semen analysis to rule out any contribution by the male partner.

We've discussed the blood supply of the testicle, the drainage of the sperm through the epididymis into the vas deferens, and the role of the prostate gland in previous chapters (See Figures 19-2, 19-3, and 19-4). Within the testicle itself, the germ cells (the term applied to cell lines dedicated to producing sperm in the male and eggs in the female) are supported on a fibrous meshwork called a stroma. The germs cells reside around the border of microscopic size tubes called the seminiferous tubules. As the sperm mature through their various stages, they move to the center of each tubule. In the final stages of maturation, they are freed from their attachments and begin the swim down the tubule. Larger tubes, called the rete testes, then connect the testicle with the epididymis (See Figure 23-1). The epididymis, if uncoiled, is approximately 18 feet long and is a single tube. This area is extremely important for maturation of the sperm and takes approximately 14 days to traverse, following a 72-day production schedule on the assembly line to manufacture the sperm. Therefore, any factors involving the previous 90

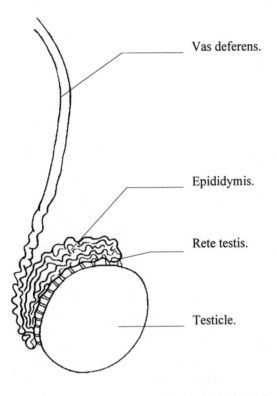

Figure 23-1: The testicle, rete testis, epididymis, and vas deferens.

days will affect the sperm ejaculated today. For this reason, generally 2 or 3 semen analyses are required for the most accuracy in diagnosis, preferably with these spaced several weeks apart.

Also within and between these microscopic tubules are two other important cell types: Sertoli Cells and Leydig Cells. Sertoli Cells are intimately involved with sperm maturation, and Leydig Cells reside in the spaces between the tubules and manufacture testosterone, the male hormone.

While extremely complex and not well understood with regards to all the factors necessary for good hearty sperm production, some general principles can be explained which will serve to help understand male infertility.

Hormones are complex chemicals produced by certain glands which then go to their " target" organ(s) producing a functional activity. The target organ or gland then produces another hormone which goes back to the original gland to regulate the production of the original hormone. This is called a feedback loop or hormonal axis. Three such hormonal loops are important in the consideration of the infertile male.

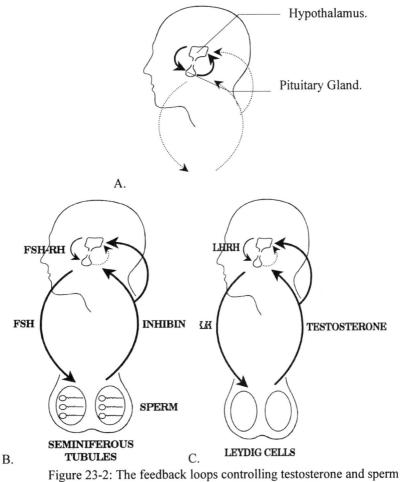

Figure 23-2: The feedback loops controlling testosterone and sperm production.

The pituitary gland, a small gland in the central portion of the brain, manufactures leutinizing hormone (LH) which travels to the testicle via the bloodstream to "turn on" the Leydig Cells of the testicle to produce the male hormone, testosterone. As the levels of testosterone increase, they are circulated by the bloodstream back through the pituitary gland to slow down the production of LH, and therefore, slow down the production of testosterone. As testosterone drops, less inhibition of the pituitary occurs and thus more LH is produced, and testosterone is once again manufactured. There obviously exists a very sensitive and finely tuned feedback loop.

The pituitary gland also produces FSH, follicle stimulating hormone, which travels through the bloodstream to the testicle, specifically acting upon a group of cells called the Sertoli Cells. These cells directly affect sperm production, and produce a hormone called Inhibin which returns to the pituitary and controls the production of further FSH. The production of testosterone has very direct affects upon the production of germ cells. The level of this hormone within the substance of the testicle is very important for this purpose.

The third feedback loop is the control of these pituitary gland functions by the hypothalamus, another small gland in the brain, by its "releasing hormones". Figure 23-2 summarizes the feedback loops controlling testosterone and sperm production.

The normal immune system at work throughout the body is not exposed to the cells destined to be sperm. We refer to the testicle as being immunologically "privileged", and any compromise of this "barrier", which is more functional than anatomic will reduce sperm production. An increased level of anti-sperm antibodies discovered either in the blood or on the sperm themselves has been found in some of these infertile men. Treatment to improve semen quality might include corticosteroid therapy.

Lastly, these problems are approached as being pre-testicular (factors acting upon a normal testicle preventing its normal function), intrinsic testicular (the testicle itself is faulty), or post-testicular (the normal factors in the production of sperm are in place but there is a blockage or problem in delivery). You now have all the necessary building blocks to have a good understanding of male infertility.

PRE-TESTICULAR FACTORS

Disorders which prevent the normal formation or function of the testicle would fall into the pre-testicular category. The easiest to understand based upon the above discussion would be problems with the glands in the brain, the pituitary or hypothalamus, which control the production of FSH and LH. Namely, pituitary tumors could shut FSH and LH off and therefore the testicles would no longer produce testosterone or sperm. Failure of normal formation or descent of the testicle could also be viewed as pre-testicular in nature, and points to the necessity of a complete history-taking by the urologist, including a review of childhood and developmental history.

INTRINSIC TESTICULAR DYSFUNCTION

A group of common conditions with an unknown etiology and for which there have been a variety of treatment regimens with variable success, this group points to the necessity of evaluating the infertile couple, as a sub-fertile male may be compensated by a super-fertile female, or vice versa. For example, if motile sperm are found on the cervical os 2 or more days after intercourse, this would be a good sign and indicate that the male is not in need of any therapy, if the other parameters of his evaluation are normal.

A flow diagram for patient selection and treatment options is depicted in Figure 23-3.

The semen analysis provides the basis for the evaluation of male infertility, yet the test is often misleading because of poor specimen handling by either the patient, the lab, or both. It is critically important to time the collection correctly. There should be 1 or 2 days of abstention prior to its collection. The specimen should represent the entire ejaculate. The highest concentration of sperm are in the first portion, just as ejaculation is started.

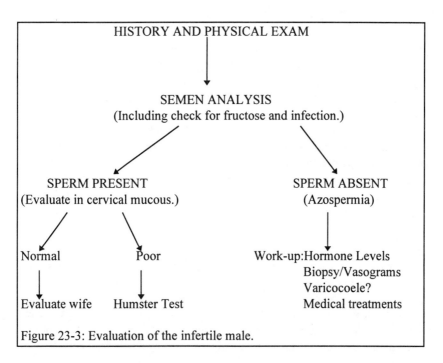

HISTORY AND PHYSICAL EXAM

SEMEN ANALYSIS
(Including check for fructose and infection.)

SPERM PRESENT
(Evaluate in cervical mucous.)

SPERM ABSENT
(Azospermia)

Normal   Poor

Evaluate wife   Humster Test

Work-up:Hormone Levels
        Biopsy/Vasograms
        Varicocoele?
        Medical treatments

Figure 23-3: Evaluation of the infertile male.

Therefore, if a "pullout method" is being used and the gentleman begins to ejaculate before he reaches the cup, the sperm counts registered by that analysis will be spuriously low. Once a good specimen is provided it should be taken promptly to the lab. While one does not need to run any red lights, the specimen should not sit on a hot dashboard while errands are run either. Generally, the specimen should be at the lab within an hour, and during that time it should be kept as close to body temperature as possible, i.e. on a cool day keep it in a jacket pocket with your hand around the specimen container to warm it. Advise the lab ahead of time, i.e. the day prior, of your approximate arrival time and don't let the receptionist let you sit in the waiting room for an hour before calling to register you. It needs to be handled in a timely fashion.

Several factors will be evaluated: volume and acidity (pH) of the ejaculate, agglutination, viscosity, and cells other than sperm, i.e. red blood cells, white blood cells, and bacteria, and sperm counts, shapes, and motility.

The best example of the intrinsic testicular dysfunction group of disorders is the varicocoele (See Scrotal Concerns, Chapter 19). As a result of the dilated veins in the scrotum, the two degree Centigrade temperature gradient between testicles and core body temperature is lost as the testicles warm. What is seen clinically is a "bag of worms" texture or appearance to the scrotum. If suspected but not appreciable by exam, an ultrasound with colorimetric doppler or thermography (temperature testing) can be diagnostic. There also may be some appreciable diminishment of testicular firmness by exam.

The classic "Stress Pattern Semen Analysis" seen with varicocoeles consists of lowered sperm counts, typically in the 10 to 20 million per cc. range, low motility, typically with less than 50% upon initial presentation, and poor morphology (shapes and sizes), usually with greater than 40% abnormal forms. Summarized, the sperm are in lower numbers with normal counts being 60 million or more per cc.; they don't seem to swim as well, with normal initial motility usually at 80% or better; and, they aren't as sleek with a variety of shapes and sizes. All of these act together to render poor semen quality. A brief note, there does **not** seem to be an association between "funny looking sperm" and "funny looking kids", that is, there is no correlation between birth defects and abnormal sperm morphology. The treatment for varicocoele is surgical and described elsewhere, semen quality improved in better than half and pregnancy achieved in 45 to 50%. Occasionally, several months after surgery, the counts may be boosted by injections of HCG which is similar in its action to LH.

The best test to assess sperm function is the sperm penetration assay, or Humster test (human sperm + hamster eggs). An in vitro (test tube) test, this assay measures the ability of the patient's sperm to penetrate hamster eggs. This is most frequently utilized to evaluate sperm function in normal males without other explainable reason for infertility.

Testicular biopsy provides a direct examination of the testicular tissue, including the seminiferous tubules and the interstitial cells. Special handling of the tissue is required and special staining procedures by the laboratory are required. Generally, the findings fall within the following groups:

1.) Normal;
2.) Maturation Arrest: in which development of the sperm occurs only up to a point and not to completion;
3.) Hypospermatogenesis: markedly lowered sperm production;
4.) Germinal Cell Aplasia: no germ cells are seen.

Other examples of intrinsic testicular factors include toxic substances ingested or exposed, i.e. steroids which diminish testosterone production; certain chemicals and insecticides to which sperm production is sensitive; and heat, i.e. hot tub or bath enthusiasts or roofers, which warm the testicles and lowers sperm production. Occasionally a small testicle results from post-pubertal mumps.

A final intrinsic testicular disease is Klinefelter's Syndrome, with an associated extra X in the chromosomal makeup (47, XXY) and very small, firm testicles. These patients usually require testosterone supplementing.

POST-TESTICULAR FACTORS

This group of disorders generally include those in which sperm production is adequate but delivery is poor. The most frequently encountered subset in this group are the patients having had a previous vasectomies. The procedure for its reversal is called a vasovasostomy. In that procedure, which generally takes between 2 and 3 hours and can be performed under the microscope utilizing local or general anesthesia. If sperm are noted in the vas deferens at the time of the surgery, nearly 90% will have sperm subsequently in the ejaculate after the surgery.

Pregnancy rates range from 30 to 70% and are highly dependent upon the time through which the patient has been vasectomized. If, for instance, the vasectomy was performed greater than 10 years prior, successful pregnancy is significantly less likely. This occurs for two reasons: additional points of blockage are possible; but more so, there is a high likelihood of anti-sperm antibodies and other factors indicating that the sperm have been barraged during their formation and/or travels through the epididymis and vas deferens. They are, therefore, not as good of swimmers and penetrators. This also is reason to ask the young patient (generally less than 26 or so) to defer on vasectomy. If he were to remarry, he is more likely to want a "second family" than the 36 year-old coming in for vasectomy consultation.

Infection and congenital deformities are less frequent causes of obstruction, yet do occur. The semen is checked for fructose to indicate its contribution by normal seminal vesicles. Previous hernia surgery or testicular surgery, even as a child, may have left one or both vas deferens occluded. The prostate gland and seminal vesicles which are responsible together for nearly 90 to 95% of the ejaculate may not have correctly formed or function or they can be harbingers of occult infections. Infections of this type are frequently asymptomatic, but may impair sperm motility, cause clumping or agglutination of sperm and affect fertility, especially if there are other factors as well, i.e., low sperm counts. An inexperienced laboratory, however, may occasionally read immature sperm forms as inflammatory cells leading to a false diagnosis of infection. Specific treatment should be directed at the organism causing the infection. In the presence of these abnormalities in the semen analysis even without a specific cultured organism, antibiotic therapy may be indicated.

Occasionally, a functional neurologic problem may exist which prevents normal ejaculation. During ejaculation, the vas deferens and sex glands contract to jettison their contents timed with a contraction of the bladder neck. This allows the ejaculate to travel out the penis. The patient may be anejaculatory, that is, nothing is ejaculated, or he may retrograde ejaculate, that is, ejaculate into the bladder. The latter is not harmful and is characterized by an extremely cloudy, clumpy urine after sexual activity. Frequently, a treatment will include a trial of alpha-adrenergic medications (cold preparations, like Sudafed® or Actifed®) to tighten the neck of the bladder allowing antegrade (normal direction) ejaculation (See Chapter 9, Bladder Basics). Additionally, the urine can be retrieved and the sperm harvested through laboratory techniques and used in the appropriate therapeutic option, i.e. assisted reproductive treatments such as intrauterine insemination. Following retroperitoneal lymph node dissection for cancer of the testicle (See Chapter 21, Male Self-Exam and Testicular Cancer), the patient may not ejaculate at all. All of the sensations associated with sexual arousal, erection, and orgasm are normal, except that little to nothing is jettisoned. Also after transurethral resection of the prostate (TURP) for prostate enlargement (See Chapter 7, Prostate Enlargement), due to a trimming away of the substance of the prostate gland and altering of the bladder neck, ejaculation is altered. Seldom is there a concern for infertility in the post-TURP patients, but the question regarding altered ejaculation is frequently asked. One is not guaranteed sterility by TURP.

Although intuitively obvious, one cannot overlook in the history the sexual practices of the couple as contributory to their infertility. Important information regarding potency (ability to sustain an erection for deep penetration and ejaculation), use of lubricants, and the couple's timing and frequency of intercourse all may be contributory and fall within the post-testicular group of disorders.

SUMMARY

In a study of more than 400 sub-fertile men, the following was the diagnoses distribution:

DIAGNOSIS	PERCENT
Varicocoele	37%
Idiopathic infertility (no known cause)	25%
Testicular failure	9%
Obstruction	6%
Cryptorchidism (undescended)	6%
Sexual dysfunction	3%
All other	14%

New therapeutic options will continue to become available to provide sufficient concentration of good quality sperm to the egg. Laboratory techniques of "sperm enhancement" in assisted reproductive techniques continue to develop. Despite all of the technology available, many of the basic questions of male component infertility remain unanswered. The importance of patience in the evaluation and treatment of this disorder, and the importance of the evaluation and treatment of the **couple** cannot be understated.

For further information write: The American Fertility Society, 2140 11th Avenue South, Suite 200, Birmingham, Alabama, 35205-2800; or call: (205) 933-8494.

CHAPTER 24

INFECTIONS OF THE URINARY TRACT

Bladder, prostate, kidney, testicle, and vaginal infections.

Infections in the urinary tract are the most common reason why a referral to a urologist occurs. They are the most common reason for prolonged hospital stays, and the most common recurring problem in the chronically ill and elderly patients. Interestingly as well, they may be the initial signal of other more significant medical problems. It's not understating the truth to say that, while urinary tract infections and vaginal infections may be looked upon as inconvenience, they cannot be overlooked with regards to their potential significance and consequence. What follows is a discussion of infections in the urinary tract based upon anatomic considerations. It's the intact patient who presents to the office or hospital, not the anatomic part. But in approaching infections in the urinary tract in this fashion, the reader should be able to appreciate the similarities, differences, and significances of infections in the different locations.

CYSTITIS: INFECTION OF THE BLADDER

Bladder infections are the most common infection site in the urinary tract. Symptoms may range from no noticeable pain or change in urinary habits to severe pain and a constant severe urge to urinate. The onset may be sudden or gradual, and generally is localized to the area just above the pubic area or into the low back, just above the buttocks. A pressure type sensation, feeling of a constant need to urinate, and a sensation of incomplete bladder emptying after urination are all common. Upon urination, the sensation that the urine is hot, or that it burns to void are voiced by the patient. Not uncommonly, there may be a change in the appearance in the urine--becoming cloudy with debris or shreds of mucous. As well, the urine may have flecks of blood, or on occasion be very bloody. Children may experience any of these symptoms and signs or simply a diffuse abdominal pain with or without fever. Small infants may simply draw up their legs with voiding or appear colicky.

The urinary tract is well equipped to protect itself from infection. These protective mechanisms include the ability to empty itself completely and in a timely fashion. The bladder becomes exposed to bacteria, the microorganisms responsible for infection, all the time. Children may experience infection from a viral cause as well. To prevent the establishment of bacterial infection, the bladder must be emptied completely and on a timely basis. Any behavior, i.e. the infrequent voider or the child who never empties because of Busy Little Girl (Boy) Syndrome (See Chapter 9, Bladder Basics and Incontinence) will predispose to infection. Additionally, any disease which would affect the ability of the bladder to empty, i.e. diabetes mellitus or a "neurogenic" bladder in the stroke patient, predisposes to infection. A basic behavior modification technique to prevent urinary tract infection is complete and timely emptying.

A second mechanism of protection is a mucous protective layer or barrier which coats the urethra and the bladder, preventing the bacteria from adhering and gaining access into the bladder. Studies have proven that women who are more prone to infection are likely to lack certain key factors in this mucous. With two groups of women giving equal attention to voiding and hygiene, this may be the predisposing factor in one group over the other for infection. As severe infection occurs, this layer may be compromised or lost. Think of the bladder in that setting as a common scrape of the skin. Touch a scrape and note that it feels sticky. Bacteria are more likely to adhere to the lining of the urethra and bladder establishing another (recurrent) or continued (chronic) infection.

The treatment then may involve not only treating the active infection, but also to provide assistance in the form of chronic or prophylactic antibiotics to prevent re-infection while the bladder is vulnerable and to allow the regeneration of the normal mucous protective barrier. This may a daily dose of antibiotic, or perhaps a dose around the time of likely inoculation, i.e. intercourse, swimming, straddle activity, exercise with tight clothing, or immersion (swimming or bathing). Some women may require this type of prevention on an ongoing basis if infection cannot be controlled or eliminated and other underlying causes of recurrent infection (discussed below) have been eliminated as contributory.

In females, recurrent infection is an indication to proceed with an evaluation. Some urologists will "spot" an otherwise healthy female, with no complicating features, her first infection. However, with even a first infection which fails to clear with appropriately chosen antibiotics based upon a urine culture and sensitivity, a second infection, or any infection (in both males and females) involving the kidneys (See Pyelonephritis, later in this chapter), most advocate a formal urologic evaluation.

In males, the additional length of the penile urethra and the prostate gland itself provide additional protection from infection. In fact, any bladder infection in a male warrants an evaluation because of the high likelihood that it is associated with an underlying anatomy problem which would predispose to infection. For instance, in an infant male there may be a condition called posterior urethral valves in which leaflets of tissue formed during the boy's development block the channel partially and prevent complete bladder emptying. In severe cases these may block enough to cause kidney failure. In the older male, a bladder cancer may present initially as an infection because the cancer does not have the mucous barrier and therefore is a sticky nidus for infection (See Chapter 14, Bladder Cancer and Blood in the Urine).

The evaluation starts with a complete history and physical examination to rule out any contribution from other health problems, i.e. steroid use for other illnesses which might retard normal defenses against infection or neurologic conditions which might inhibit the bladder's ability to empty. The urinalysis is the chemical analysis (usually by dip-sticking of the urine with chemical strips) and microscopic analysis which will render suspicion of infection. The urine culture is the incubation of the urine for bacterial growth, and the additional testing of different antibiotics against those bacteria to select the appropriate antibiotic treatment is called the sensitivity.

Formal testing includes the IVP (intravenous pyelogram), an xray test in which contrast or dye (although the term dye is inaccurate because the liquid used, while visible on xray, is colorless to the eye) is administered into the vein, usually of the arm, and filtered by the kidneys during which time xrays are taken of the abdomen. This will demonstrate any anatomic problems of the kidneys, i.e. certain types of infection-ladened kidney stones (See Chapter 17A and 17C, Kidney Stones, Causes, and Prevention) or blockages to the drainage of the kidneys which would predispose the kidneys to infection (See Chapter 16, Kidney Lumps). Also, this test allows us to assess the degree of kidney damage, if any, from prior infections by demonstrating scarring of the kidneys. If there is concern regarding contrast allergy, kidney function to handle the filtration of the contrast or dye, or in children in whom we try to limit the exposure to xray, a kidney ultrasound may suffice. In this test, painless sound waves are bounced off of the kidneys to give us an image of the kidneys' architecture. This test does not assess kidney function, however, and therefore the IVP still remains the gold standard of the evaluation.

If indicated, and especially appropriate in children with infections, an additional xray test called the voiding cystourethrogram (or VCUG for short) may be ordered. In this test, the bladder is filled with contrast through a catheter which has been placed into the bladder. The patient then has xrays taken as urination occurs. This test allows direct visualization of the emptying of the bladder and assures that no urine is allowed to reflux or yo-yo back up to the kidneys during urination. In the condition called vesicoureteral reflux, as the pressure rises in the bladder during urination, urine is pushed back up the ureter (the tube connecting the kidney down to the bladder on each side) on one or both sides. Normally the anatomy prevents this. However, what reflux does is prevent complete emptying because of that volume which is refluxed and therefore predisposing to infection; and if infection does occur, it provides a direct route for that infection to access the kidneys.

Let's digress for a moment and discuss reflux. The principle factor which prevents urine from going back up to the kidneys during voiding is the length of the ureter as it traverses through the wall of the bladder (See Figure 24-1). Hold a pencil between your straightened fingers. The length traversing through your fingers is only the width of your fingers. Now tip the pencil relative to the fingers at an angle, note that the length of the pencil now traverses through your fingers is considerably longer. The longer that distance, the less likely reflux is to occur. Any surgery for reflux does exactly this--it reconstructs this length to prevent reflux.

The decision to correct this congenital problem is based upon:

      1.) its unlikelihood to resolve spontaneously (many will correct with growth);
      2.) the failure to control infection through the use of"suppression" antibiotics while waiting for growth to occur;
      3.) indications on xray of kidney damage while on suppression antibiotics; or
      4.) or failure to correct reflux by puberty.

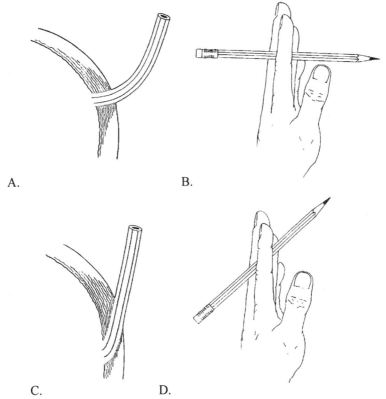

A.   B.

C.   D.

Figure 24-1: The relationship of the ureter and the bladder.

Now back to the evaluation of bladder infections: A cystoscopy (look in the bladder) is also in order to assess, by direct visualization, any anatomic problems in the bladder which would predispose to infection. For instance with reflux as discussed above, the ureteral orifices (the holes in the bladder through which the urine from the kidneys is expulsed) have a very characteristic appearance with different degrees of reflux. This appearance may allow a prognosis for spontaneous resolution to be given. In children cystoscopy usually requires general anesthesia. Direct visualization would also allow the assessment for any bladder lesions, i.e. cancer or chronic infection, which would predispose to recurrent infection. In older men, the degree of prostate enlargement and obstruction of the bladder outlet can also be assessed (See Prostate Enlargement, Chapter 7). Urodynamics, or studies of the tone and emptying of the bladder, may also be indicated (See Chapter 9, Bladder Basics).

Treatments are obviously directed at any underlying factor which may be the cause, i.e. elimination of an infected kidney stone, medical treatment or surgery for reflux, or treatment of prostate enlargement in an older gentleman. In the absence of any predisposing anatomic conditions, specific antibiotic treatment directed at culture-specified infection is important as are good emptying habits on a complete and timely basis.

Use of prophylactic antibiotics, in selected patients (as discussed above), is indicated again assuming there are no other identified contributory factors. The best antibiotics used in this setting are nearly 100% absorbed in the upper intestine (therefore the colon and rectum where the bacteria causing infection originate never have the opportunity to be exposed to them and to develop resistance), they are almost 100% filtered on first pass through the kidneys (which means that they attain very high levels in the urine), and in being so completely filtered by the kidneys they do not accumulate in other secretions of the body, i.e. vaginal secretions, and therefore are not prone to cause yeast infections.

For the patient with recurring infection, the negative evaluation can only serve as reassurance of the absence of any underlying problem. With attentiveness to voiding habits, identifying factors which might predispose to infection, and through carefully orchestrated evaluation and treatment, hopefully the vicious cycle of recurrence can be broken.

PROSTATITIS: INFECTION OF THE PROSTATE GLAND

Infections of the prostate will be discussed in Chapter 25 entitled "Prostatitis". In adult males, the prostate gland is the most usual source of infection by preventing complete emptying and by becoming infected itself within the substance of the gland. In severe cases, the infection may gain access into the bloodstream either directly through the prostate itself or by tracking up to the kidneys (See Pyelonephritis, later in this chapter) rendering an illness of even life-threatening severity.

EPIDIDYMORCHITIS: INFECTION OF THE TESTICLE AND EPIDIDYMIS

Infections involving the testicle and its associated structures including the epididymis, are discussed in Chapter 20 entitled "The Acute Scrotum". These infections have generally tracked from the urethra (tube connecting the bladder to the outside), and they too may involve the bladder, particularly if caused by bacteria.

PYELONEPHRITIS: INFECTION OF THE KIDNEY

Prior to the antibiotic era, infections of the kidney were more commonly caused by a transport of an infection from elsewhere, i.e. an infected joint or pneumonia, to the kidney through the bloodstream. With more aggressive treatments for infections of all kinds, this route of spread now represents less than 5% of all infections of the kidneys.

More commonly, infections ascend the tubes (ureters) connecting the kidneys to the bladder. The classic triad of presentation is fever, flank pain, and pyuria (pus in the urine under the microscope). Any fever associated with a urinary tract infection is assumed to be a pyelonephritis. This means that the treatment will be more aggressive and prolonged. Also, it means that even a first urinary tract infection should be evaluated subsequent to successful treatment of the active infection because of the high likelihood of discovering an underlying cause, i.e. a specific anatomic problem, which would predispose to recurrence of infection. As more aggressive antibiotics become available in tablet form, more patients with pyelonephritis are treated in the outpatient (at home) setting. Any state of general debilitation, severe illness associated with nausea/vomiting or dehydration, or associated medical conditions which would retard response to infection are all indications to treat this potentially life-threatening infection in the hospital setting.

As described above, any pyelonephritic episode warrants a full urologic evaluation once the acute infection is treated and the urine has been sterilized of infection.

VAGINITIS

Many complaints seemingly referable to the bladder may be, in fact, symptoms of vaginal infection. Therefore, urologists should be concerned with and well versed in the diagnosis and treatment of the different causes of vaginitis. If an incorrect diagnosis is made of a urinary tract infection while, in fact, the patient has a vaginal infection, the bladder and urethral symptoms of irritation may be worsened as antibiotic therapy may be a contributing cause to the vaginitis in the first place. This occurs because the antibiotics, selected to treat a bladder infection (or any infection, for that matter), also kill the normal bacteria which live in the vagina. These bacteria normally "out-compete" with the yeast, which also normally exist in the vagina in limited numbers. Once the bactereria are eliminated by an antibiotic, the yeast are allowed to grow completely unrestricted as they are not sensitive to the antibiotics and have an unlimited source of nutrients available in the vaginal secretions. This overgrowth results in irritation and a foul discharge. Vaginitis has been estimated to account for up to 50% of a private gynecologic practice and approximately 33% of complaints from women attending sexually transmitted disease clinics.

Typical symptoms include vaginal discharge (of varying degrees, colors, and odors), vaginal and vulvar (female external genitals) irritation, dysuria (painful urination), and dysparunia (painful intercourse). Accurate diagnosis is best made by assessing the color and texture of the discharge, determining its acidity, and examining the discharge microscopically--one observation and two simple office laboratory tests.

Trichomoniasis (or "Trich"), Candidiasis (or Yeast"), and Nonspecific Vaginitis (or NSV) are the most common types. With Trichomoniasis, the discharge is usually gray or yellow-green and is generally thin in consistency to frothy. The trichomonad is usually easily seen under the microscope, and the treatment is metronidazole. With Candidiasis, the yeast is usually seen easily under the microscope. The discharge is usually white or yellow-white, the consistency is curd-like or cheesy, and the treatment is a whole host of antifungals from which to choose, now over-the-counter. Nonspecific Vaginitis is often a diagnosis of exclusion as no causative organisms are seen under the microscope or the patient has failed previous treatment for a presumed cause. A malodorous discharge which may be quite light and thin suggests this diagnosis. Treatment for the Gardenella vaginalis infection causing NSV is metronidazole or ampicillin.

Regarding treatment of the male sexual partners, with Trichomoniasis, treatment of the male sexual partner simultaneously is indicated. With yeast infections and NSV, treatment of the male is more debatable. Studies indicate that yeast is four times more likely to be present on the penis of partners of women who suffer recurrent infection. There is no clinical evidence supporting the treatment of asymptomatic male sexual partners of women who are experiencing their initial yeast infection. Therefore, in monogamous relationships with recurrence of either yeast or Nonspecific Vaginitis, treatment of the asymptomatic male sexual partner is reasonable.

Two other principles are critically important, particularly now that many of the products to treat vaginal infections are available as over-the-counter products. There should not be hesitation to seek medical opinion if there is any doubt regarding the diagnosis, as delay could lead to more serious consequences of an infection and contribute to further spread if condom protection or abstinence is not practiced until the infection is cleared. Secondly, the association of recurrent infection with sexual activity may lead not only to less satisfactory sexual activity because of the anxiety caused by the dysparunia (painful intercourse) but also to less lubrication and relaxation of the vagina thus contributing to more trauma to the vagina and more pain, thereby completing the cycle of problematic activity.

For more information on infections of the urinary tract write or call: National Kidney and Urologic Diseases Information Clearinghouse (NKUDIC), Box NKUDIC, Bethesda, MD., 20892; (301) 468-6345.

CHAPTER 25

PROSTATITIS

Inflammation of the prostate gland.

Inflammation of the prostate can be very confusing and frustrating. This is to the urologist what low back pain is to the orthopedist or neurosurgeon in that they tend to be a chronic or recurring and can be extremely prolonged in their treatment to see improvement. This understanding right from the very outset will help the patient who has multiple recurrences or who, three months into treatment, is still having good days and bad days to deal with his illness.

The symptoms can be confusing and not immediately recognized as associated with the urinary tract, or specifically to the prostate gland. Prostatititis is a great mimicker. By virtue of its location deep within the pelvis and surrounded by several sensitive structures, irritation in the prostate gland can transmit that irritation to the structures which surround it or which attach to it rendering a whole host of symptoms.

Patients may experience a low back pain which they associate with a musculoskeletal strain. They may experience a deep, gnawing ache in the perineum (that area between the base of the scrotum and the anus). They may experience deep pain in the rectum, particularly during defecation (the act of having a bowel movement), as the bowel movement compresses the prostate in its passage through the low rectum. They may experience orchalgia (aching in the testicles, one or both) resulting from the connection of the testicle to the prostate by the vas deferens. Occasionally they may experience an associated infection in the testicles (See Epididymorchitis discussed in Chapter 20 entitled The Acute Scrotum.) as a result of the infection tracking up this connecting route.

They may experience severe pain either shortly before ejaculation as the prostate gland "gears up" during sexual activity, or they may have post-ejaculatory pain--pain after ejaculation. They may have no pain but notice a change in the color, texture, or volume of the ejaculate. Recall that the prostate is responsible for approximately 25 to 50% by volume of what's ejaculated. Along with the prostate gland, the two seminal vesicles, which attach to the prostate like rabbit ears to its head, are involved in up to 80% of prostate infections. Because of the seminal vesicles' manufacturing of an additional 50% or so of the ejaculate, not unexpectedly, infections of the prostate gland and/or seminal vesicles can be a contributor to male component infertility by impairing sperm motility (See Male Infertility, Chapter 23).

Most commonly, however, the patient with prostatitis experiences changes in his urinary habits and pain associated with the bladder. The symptoms are a result of the configuration of the prostate as it surrounds the neck of the bladder like a collar and by virtue of the configuration of the prostate gland as adjoining that area of the bladder with the highest concentration of nerves directing its activity. Again, think of the prostate as a donut. With infection, the donut not only swells and becomes larger, but the hole in the donut shrinks, resulting in higher pressures necessary to urinate. This may cause irritation symptoms of burning with urination or a sense of not emptying well, in addition to a slowed stream from the tightening of the aperture. Because of the irritation of the nerves in the neck of the bladder, the bladder may misinterpret the nerves firing resulting in a continuous need to urinate (See Figure 6-2, Chapter 6). The inflammation of the bladder may yield an aching or discomfort across the lower abdomen, particularly right above the pubic bone (the bone at the lower border of the abdomen above the genitalia). On occasion, the patient with prostatitis may have no complaints with the diagnosis made by an abnormal rectal exam with swelling noted, by abnormal urinalysis noting red blood cells (microscopic hematuria) or white blood cells (pyuria), or occasionally the passage of visible blood.

On rare occasion, particularly in the older patient or the patient with compromised ability to combat infection, i.e. with diabetes mellitus, malnourishment, cancer, or other challenging diseases, the patient presents with a fulminant, overwhelming infection. A result of a raging infection with a pouring of the infection itself and the toxins of the infecting bacteria into the bloodstream, these patients are extremely ill--with death a likely possibility if left untreated within the next few hours. These patients may have high fevers, loss of consciousness or confusion, drop in blood pressure, and frequently urinary retention from the tense swollen prostate completely obstructing the bladder outlet. Even a rectal exam with prostatic massage is not indicated in these patients as this may invoke a further spray of infection and toxins into the system. These patients require immediate hospitalization with aggressive antibiotic therapy, fluid treatment, and instrumentation only if absolutely necessary, i.e. a catheter to drain the bladder.

The history given by the the more typical patient will lead to a suspicion of prostatitis. Suspicion then would lead to a rectal exam.The prostate will often be swollen and tender. Usually approximating the texture of the mound of tissue at the base of our thumb on the palm of the hand (thenar eminence), the prostate will swell to 2 to 3 times its normal size and assume a texture which is more spongy--referred to as boggy.

The diagnosis is assisted by collecting serial specimens in which the urine is fractioned in order to localize the infection. By collecting specimens in stages (first 10 ml. voided, second 200 ml., prostatic massage specimen, and 10 ml. post-prostatic massage urine), bacteria counts from the urethra, midstream bladder urine, and prostate expressate can be compared. The urinalysis may be entirely normal, or may be only mildly abnormal with only a few inflammatory cells (white blood cells) seen under the microscope. However, examination of the first 10 to 20 ml. of urine passed after the examination of the prostate (or the examination of secretions expressed from the penis after a "massage " of the prostate) may show considerably more white blood cells (WBC's). The more severe cases will usually demonstrate WBC's in both the voided and post prostatic massage urines.

TREATMENT

Every patient with prostatitis should be made aware of the chronicity and recurrent nature of the illness. This will help to diffuse the frustration which frequently is experienced by the otherwise healthy, young man who seemingly "can't shake this thing".

Important for the urologist is the recognition and separation of the different types of prostatitis to direct specific treatment. Four main groups include:

     1.) acute bacterial prostatitis
     2.) chronic bacterial prostatitis
     3.) non-bacterial prostatitis
     4.) prostatodynia (chronic prostate gland pain)

The infection, if bacterial in origin, is often attributable to the gram negative bacteria, the same group causing bladder infections in women. The difficulty in treatment is that the substance of the prostate gland becomes embedded with infection and becomes very difficult to clear. Many of the body's normal defenses are inactivated because of the chemical environment which normally exists in the prostate, and many of the very good antibiotics either do not penetrate the substance of the prostate gland well or are chemically inactive there. Occasionally, small abscesses (microabscesses: pockets of pus and debris large enough to be seen only under the microscope) contribute to the inability to be readily cleared and to recurrence. Also, on occasion small stones which accumulate in the prostate gland even in the uninfected patient, will secondarily become infected and lead to recurrence. In its worst cases, prostatitis can proceed on to frank abscess formation which requires surgical drainage.

With the diagnosis of acute or chronic bacterial prostatitis made, treatment consists of appropriately chosen antibiotics for prolonged lengths of treatment. The quinolones are currently the best group of antibiotics because of their coverage and their ability to permeate the prostate. The duration of treatment is frequently for up to a month initially, with a refill necessary if any symptoms persist or inflammation is still readily apparent on rectal exam. Frequently, a non-steroidal antiinflammatory is teamed with the antibiotic for the first several days of treatment, mainly to quiet symptoms from the inflammation as the antibiotic has a chance to kill the bacteria causing the infection along with the patient's immune system. I also believe this lessens the likelihood of prolonged symptoms, called prostatodynia or chronic prostate pain, even after the infection has been addressed. If infection still is apparent, chronic antibiotics, i.e. a single dose a day of a trimethoprim/sulfa combination, may be utilized. While this group is frequently used as first-line therapy, in this setting it is more to prevent resurgence or reinoculation as the patient's own defenses mend the vulnerable prostate gland.

On occasion, a formal urologic evaluation including an intravenous pyelogram xray (IVP) and cystoscopy is suggested in stubborn cases to rule out any unknown factors which may be contributing to the inability to be cleared or to the cause for recurrence, i.e. a bladder tumor or stones. Most often this fails to reveal any additional problems, but it does reassure the patient and the urologist that no stones (or cancers) have been left unturned.

Very important to the resolution of symptoms is the behavior modification of the patient. Irritants must be eliminated and include: caffeine (coffee, tea, and pop), nicotine, spicy foods, chocolate, nuts, alcohol, and stress. It's always amazing to me that a gentleman would drop $100 for antibiotics (and complain about their cost), but refuse to give up his 5 or 6 cups of coffee every morning. I suggest complete elimination of these irritants during the acute phase, and elimination of excesses for several weeks after marked improvement has been achieved. Much like salt does not cause the wound but certainly will inflame it, these do not cause the problem, but they certainly do worsen the symptoms.

Prolonged symptoms after resolved prostatitis (prostatodynia) are frequently a result of "spasm" either of the neck of the bladder, particularly the spirally-oriented muscle which constitutes the internal sphincter. In spasm, it may not relax adequately to allow good urination or may be a continued source of a deep, internal aching pain. This is treated with medications previously described to relax this muscle to improve urine flow, i.e. terazosin or prazosin (See Chapter 7, Prostate Enlargement). Additionally, patients may experience pain from spasm of the external sphincter, the sheet of muscle upon which the prostate sits, like an apple on a table, and which clips the urethra to prevent incontinence until it totally relaxes during the act of urination. Transmitted irritation from prolonged prostatitis can cause spasm and pain. The treatment here is a muscle relaxant, the best choice being diazepam or one of its cousins.

One final word, particularly important in the patient older than age 50, is the follow-up exam for a rectal check performed upon a totally uninflammed prostate. This is necessary to rule out any occult prostate malignancy. The active infection and swelling can obscure a lump. Therefore, re-exam is the rule, and several weeks to even a few months after the storm has been quieted, a PSA (prostatic specific antigen) is in order to check for malignancy not detectable by exam. Done in the context of active infection, the PSA will uniformly be elevated. Therefore, there is a need to delay ordering the test to allow for complete resolution of the post-infection inflammation. It would not need to be repeated if it had been performed within the last 6 to 12 months and was normal.

CHAPTER 26

VENEREAL (SEXUALLY TRANSMITTED) DISEASES

Sexually transmitted diseases.

Disease obtained through exposure during sexual activity is termed venereal disease. While we are barraged with the message of the dangers of unprotected sexual activity, in part because of the AIDS awareness programs and the fact that the ultimate price (death) is paid by the patient with AIDS, these diseases have often been the source of a snicker by many but the scourge for those who have contracted them. Because of the pervasiveness of these diseases and the limitations of human nature demonstrated throughout history in preventing their spread, these diseases have become a national health priority.

URETHRITIS (GONOCOCCAL)

Infection of the urethra with a bacteria called Neisseria gonorrhea results in a painful urethra with a foul discharge. The 2 to 5 days of incubation means that the symptoms will not occur for that time and may allow the infection to be given to other sexual partners. During the time of incubation, the bacteria are multiplying in the mucous-secreting glands which normally line the urethra. These then drain to release the purulent discharge or may go on to develop frank abscesses, or pockets of pus, which require surgical drainage.

The prostate gland and epididymis are rarely (less than 2%) involved. In males, up to 30% may have associated throat (pharyngeal) infections in the homosexual population, occurring only 10% in heterosexuals. The risk of acquiring gonococcal urethritis for a man after a single exposure to an infected woman is 20% and increases to 60% to 80% following 4 exposures. Conversely, the prevalence of infection in women after sexual contact with men who have gonococcal urethritis has been reported to be 50% to 90%. In rare cases, the infection may be disseminated through the bloodstream yielding pustular skin lesions, inflammation of joints, and fever. Over the long term in males, even if optimally and promptly treated, stricture disease of the urethra may occur. This scarring of the urethra may take up to 15 to 18 years after the infection to develop and may result in difficult urination by its constriction of the urethral caliber.

In females, the cervix is more commonly involved than the urethra, anal canal, or throat. 50% of salpingitis, inflammation of the Fallopian tubes which bridge the ovaries to the uterus, is caused by gonorrhea. Not only does this sometimes lead to an acute exploratory surgery to evaluate and treat the cause of an extremely painful "surgical" abdomen, it may also lead to sterility or increased likelihood of subsequent tubal pregnancy from the resultant scarring after the infection is healed. One episode of salpingitis leads to approximately a 15% sterility rate. Three such episodes will render the woman approximately 75% likely of being sterile. Yet, up to 80% of women with gonorrhea are without symptoms.

The diagnosis of gonorrhea is made from a microscopic examination and culture of the discharge. And while the treatments vary based upon the severity of the presentation, i.e. urethritis alone or in combination with salpingitis also taking into consideration the patients medical history particularly any drug allergies, various antibiotics are at the physician's disposal. Re-culture to assure complete treatment is necessary.

Strict protection during sexual activity is advised. The sexual contacts must be notified of their potential infection and need to be checked. The case is recorded with the Centers for Disease Control (CDC), and AIDS testing and counseling are appropriate. In 1990, more than 700,000 cases of gonorrhea were reported to the Centers for Disease Control and Prevention. Associated with antibiotic treatment is treatment for a possible second venereal exposure at the same time gonorrhea was contracted, namely post-gonococcal, nonspecific urethritis discussed further below.

GENITAL ULCER DISEASE

An ulcer is an open sore resembling a small crater. Syphilis, caused by the organism Treponema pallidum, is contacted through a break in the skin or mucous membranes, with the risk of acquiring the disease approaching 60% after sexual contact with an infected individual. The primary lesion, called a chancre, then appears generally around 3 weeks later and consists of a painless ulcer with a raised edge. There may be swollen lymph nodes in the groins. If not recognized or treated, a systemic illness (involving the whole body) will manifest including a characteristic rash, swollen lymph nodes, tender joints, and liver and/or kidney involvement. Latent syphilis may occur with involvement of the central nervous system.

Microscopic examination will demonstrate the Treponema spirochete, and serologic testing (that portion of the blood without the cells) will be positive for diagnosis. Penicillin remains the treatment of choice.

An additional ulcer lesion is Chancroid, and Hemophilus ducreyi is the organism responsible. The incubation period is usually 4 to 7 days with a deep painful genital ulcer apparent. Most lesions occur within the redundant foreskin (prepuce), on the frenulum (the web on the underside of the penis in its center), or on the coronal sulcus (the groove around the head). Treatment is with ceftriaxone injection.

NONSPECIFIC URETHRITIS

Approximately 80% of all urethritis in male college students is nonspecific urethritis. The pain is usually less than that seen with gonorrhea, frequently being only an awareness of the urethra or a slight burning upon urination. The discharge is less foul than gonorrhea, frequently being only a clear, mucousy type, and frequently symptoms resolve on their own yet the infection remains with the patient, capable of infecting others. In healthy, asymptomatic male military recruits, 10% positive cultures for one or both organisms generally held accountable for nonspecific urethritis, Chlamydia trichomatis and Ureaplasma urealyticum, are reported. The organisms are difficult to culture, and therefore treatment is most commonly based upon a clinical diagnosis rather than a positive test. It is important to have the sexual partner treated as well to prevent "ping-pong" back-and-forth contamination.

In males, up to 40% may progress on to an epididymorchitis (See Chapter 20, The Acute Scrotum), or inflammation of the epididymis rendering an exquisitely tender, swollen testicle. In addition to antibiotic therapy, scrotal elevation, ice packs, and often a nonsteroidal antiinflammatory, i.e. ibuprofen, are teamed in the treatment.

With nonspecific urethritis, tetracycline is the drug of choice, and the sexual partner should be treated as well. Even silent infection or potential infection should be treated in females to prevent its spread unknowingly to other sexual partners and to preclude the risk for the development of salpingitis (inflammation of the Fallopian Tubes). Erythromycin can be tried if the tetracycline fails. Condom protection should be used while treatment is underway, and always used in any other than a monogamous relationship.

The estimated incidence of chlamydial infections is 3 to 4 million annually.

VENEREAL WARTS

Condyloma accuminata are venereal warts caused by the transmission sexually of a virus, the human papillomavirus (HPV), which results in the formation of wart growth on the skin of the genitalia, both male and female. Women, while forming warts on the external surfaces, may have lesions on the cervix or vaginal wall. It is now not disputed that HPV is associated with the development of cervical cancer in women. While men generally form lesions on the penis and within the escutcheon (pubic hair), rarely they may form lesions down the urethra. Generally in extensive cases, particularly those involving the glans penis (head of the penis), lesions down the urethra may be found and treated by urethroscopy (similar instrumentation to cystoscopy, but only the urethra is viewed).

The incubation period is varied and may be months, but approximately two-thirds of sex partners with genital warts will develop lesions within a 3-month incubation period.

While all lesions may be treated, it remains important to reexamine the patient quarterly for a minimum of one year during which time condom protection is required. Oral sexual activity may result in laryngeal seeding and is to be discouraged as well. Reexamination requires not only inspection, but the use of an acetic acid application and examination using magnification looking for any "acetowhite" lesions which indicate viral infection and the potential for condyloma growth. Subclinical HPV infection may be present in up to 10% of asymptomatic males and females. Critically important is that both sexual partners are checked as well with similar techniques to prevent the risk of "ping-ponging" the infection back and forth.

The treatment options include topical medications which destroy the virally infected tissues, i.e. podophyllin, trichloroacetic acid (TCA), 5-fluorouracil (5-FU); injection, i.e. interferon injected 3 times per week for 3 weeks; surgical excision (generally reserved for extensive cases); and laser therapy, i.e. CO2 laser or Nd:YAG laser, which is the treatment of choice. Laser therapy is used for external lesions, but it can also be used through the urethroscope for treatment of urethral lesions. Laser energy is less destructive to the surrounding tissues and therefore is less painful and less likely to scar extensively (See Figure 14-3).

The need for follow-up checks cannot be understated, but assuming good follow-up for both sexual partners in a monogamous setting and using appropriate precautions with use of a condom and limiting sexual partners, a nearly 90% cure rate can be offered in one treatment. In other than a monogamous setting and without use of proper protection, no such assurances can be made for this disease which increased its incidence more than 450% between 1973 and 1988.

HERPES

A blister-type lesion, or cluster of blisters, occurring in the oral and genital areas results from the infection with one or more of six different viruses. The lesions may be preceded by pain, itching, or even a discharge, and result from an incubation period ranging between one and 45 days, but generally less than one week subsequent to the sexual exposure. A noninfected female exposed to an infected male has 80% to 90% risk of developing genital herpes. Asymptomatic infection is nearly 50% and rate of transmission in this group is highly dependent upon the presence of active lesions (visible lesions which are either in blister form or weeping shallow ulcers). Healing takes approximately 2 to 3 weeks for the first infection, during which time sexual activity, particularly unprotected, is to be avoided. Treatment consists of acyclovir, either oral or topical, to reduce the time of active virus shedding and to speed wound healing. Even so, the average rate of recurrence is 5 episodes per year, occurring especially during times of stress or lowered body defenses, i.e. during or after a severe bout of another infection like influenza.

One additional note on active herpes virus in the pregnant female. If labor occurs and the women is thought to be at risk for actively-shedding herpes lesions, the child should be delivered by Caeserian section to bypass the vaginal canal where the infection exists. If the neonate is exposed to the virus, the child is at significant risk for the development of a life-threatening infection with the virus or possibly a severe infection of the eyes which could result in blindness.

AIDS

Acquired Immunodeficiency Syndrome (AIDS) is discussed Chapter 27.

HEPATITIS B

Sexual transmission remains the most common route of transmission for this form of viral hepatitis. Particularly at risk are heterosexual men and women with multiple sexual partners, homosexual men, and sex partners of intravenous drug users. Vaccination is available for those at high risk.

The following indications for the use of the Hepatitis B vaccine have been recommended by the Immunization Practices Advisory Committee (ACIP) of the Centers for Disease Control:

1.) Health-care workers;
2.) Patients and staffs of institutions for the mentally retarded;
3.) Hemodialysis patients;
4.) Homosexually active men;
5.) Users of illicit injectable drugs;
6.) Recipients of certain blood products, i.e. clotting factor concentrates;
7.) Household and sexual contacts of Hepatitis B virus carriers;
8.) Other contacts of Hepatitis B virus carriers, i.e. i.e. classroom contacts of deinstitutionalized, mentally retarded carriers. Casual contacts are at minimal risk of acquiring Hepatitis B;
9.) Special high-risk populations depending upon public health considerations;
10.) Inmates of long-term correctional facilities;
11.) Heterosexually active persons with multiple partners;
12.) International travelers.

MOLLUSCUM CONTAGIOSUM (MCV)

A small waxy lesion anywhere on the skin surfaces, generally painless, may be the result of the virus Poxviridae. These need not be sexually acquired, and among infants and children in whom it is more common, are not the product of sexual transmission. These generally grow slowly and are self-limited, resolving spontaneously. Silver nitrate, phenol, and cryotherapy (freezing) have all been described for removal of lesions.

TRICHOMONIASIS

Approximately 2.5 to 3 million women will contract Trichomoniasis this year. Generally women who are infected with Trichomonas vaginalis experience a profuse, foul vaginal discharge. Men, although less likely to have asymptomatic infection, will have complaints of burning and a discharge. Both sexual partners should be examined and treated. The diagnosis is made by examining the discharge under the microscope for the very characteristic organisms. Treatment is with metronidazole which has the side effect of severe nausea and vomiting if alcohol is also ingested.

LICE AND MITES

Intimate contact allows transmission of human lice, causing irritation by the lice and eggs, and is treated with Kwell® applied to the affected areas.

Scabies is an irritation caused by the burrowing of the mite. Treatment is the application of Lidane®.

SUMMARY

Any concern regarding a genital lesion or discharge should be brought promptly to the attention of a physician to provide early and accurate diagnosis and treatment. Not only lessening the discomfort currently experienced by the patient, early treatment can prevent long term problems (for example, infertility, loss of testicle or tube/ovary, adverse pregnancy outcomes, and potential genital neoplasms) and minimize the risk of spread of disease to others. Alternate sexual practices, i.e. oral sexual practices, do not eliminate the risk of alternate routes of infection and spread. Ultimately, the use of condom for protection of both sexual partners is necessary. However, even with condom protection, there must be proper precautions with the proper storage and use if successful prevention of unwanted pregnancy and disease is to be reasonably assured. These include:

1.) Use a new latex condom for each act of intercourse;
2.) Put on the condom before any sexual contact;
3.) Make sure no air is trapped inside the condom;
4.) Use only water-based lubricants as oil-based lubricants can

cause the condom to dissolve;

       5.) Immediately withdraw after sex, holding the condom to prevent slippage;

       6.) Properly store new condoms at a reasonable temperature; a man's wallet does not qualify.

Specifically regarding the HIV (AIDS): one study of 89 latex condoms did have 29 which "leaked" for the HIV-sized particles. The pores in the latex are approximately 10 times smaller than sperm, thereby preventing their "escape" or that of similar-sized organisms causing most infections. However, the AIDS virus is approximately **50 times smaller** than these inherent pores in the latex fabric. Therefore, one may be subject to a 30% failure rate for protection from HIV by strict reliance upon a latex condom.

In summary, with any relationship other than one of commitment and fidelity, one continues to be at risk for being infected with a venereal disease.

CHAPTER 27

AIDS: ACQUIRED IMMUNODEFICIENCY SYNDROME

Acquired Immunodeficiency Syndrome.

The Acquired Immunodeficiency Syndrome (AIDS) was first described in the early 1980's. No disease has captured more attention than AIDS. While the attention has brought awareness, unfortunately it cast political and ethical shadowing upon a disease even as our scientific understanding was in its infancy. By the end of 1991, approximately 1.5 million Americans alone were infected, 270,000 AIDS cases had occurred, and 179,000 of these had died--100,000 in the last 2 years. The prevalence of HIV infection (that is, infection in the absence of symptoms) has ranged from 0 to 1.2 per 100 persons in groups without identified high risk.

An infectious cause was suggested because of the clustering of initial cases around sexual contacts and blood products. By 1983 a retrovirus (a member of the lentivuruses so named because months or years may ensue between the infection and the onset of symptoms) had been identified and has come to be known as immunodeficiency virus type 1 (HIV 1). Subsequently, a related virus was identified in humans from Western African and has been termed HIV 2. Other viruses are now being investigated resulting in the AIDS syndrome, including non-HIV causes.

Once infected, the individual develops antibodies (or an immune response) which do not protect but do provide the ability to be tested for the infection by a blood test. The ELISA, or enzyme-linked immunosorbent assay for you eponym buffs, with a sensitivity and specificity of greater than 95%, is the test used. If positive, a second equally specific test called the Western Blot is used. It is possible to test negative during a "window" prior to the development of HIV antibodies, estimated to be three months or less. High risk exposures require interim protection and re-testing.

It is the profound compromise of our immunity, particularly what is called our cell-mediated immunity, that is characteristic of AIDS and ultimately leads to the demise of the infected person rendering conditions which are direct manifestations of the inability to combat malignancy or even the commonest of infections, called "opportunistic infections". This wide range of presentations, from silent carrier to fulminantly infected or overwhelmed with malignancy, led to confusion initially. Infected patients do have a chronic progressive disease that ultimately will lead to significantly impaired immunity and death. Remember, these are slow viruses. The rate of progression to symptoms appears to be approximately 4% to 10% per year of infection. AIDS is the last, and most dramatic, stage of the infection--when the patient can no longer control the infections and malignancies that rarely occur in "normal" individuals.

The means of transmission of the virus are three: direct sexual contact, perinatal transmission, and exposure to blood or blood products. There is no proof that HIV can be contracted from other sources, i.e. casual contact, human or insect bites, fecal contamination, or contamination by food or water.

The best studies indicate that large numbers of sexual partners and sexual acts involving anal intercourse unprotected by condoms increase the likelihood of infection with HIV. Lack of a condom, being uncircumcised, and having ulcerative lesions (open sores) on the penis all increase risk. However, even condom use does not guarantee protection against potential infection by sexual transmission (See Chapter 26, Venereal Disease). Transmission may occur between homosexual and heterosexual persons. Between 1986 and 1991, the percentage of AIDS patients who acquired HIV through homosexual transmission declined from 65% to 52.7%.

Children can acquire HIV through sexual exposure or transfusion of blood or blood products, but approximately 80% contract the disease from an IV drug-using mother.

Intravenous drug users constitute the second largest category of AIDS patients--increased in likelihood by extensive drug use, needle-sharing, and the use of crack cocaine.

Regarding the risk of contracting the HIV from blood or blood products, i.e. "pooled" clotting factors from a number of donors, results have demonstrated a VIRTUAL ELIMINATION OF NEW HIV FROM BLOOD TRANSFUSIONS, since the institution of screening of all units of blood or organs donated since the spring of 1985. Those at risk for or positive for HIV can utilize the self-deferral option provided by blood centers in order to eliminate the risk of inadvertent transmission and to protect their medical confidentiality, i.e. in the setting of a company blood drive. The number of infected units being transfused is estimated to be 70 to 460 per year in the U.S. for a risk of 1 in 40,000 to 1 in 250,000 transfused units. The problem of potential transmission of HIV by "pooled" units for blood factor concentrates has been virtually eliminated through the development of heat treatment.

Approximately 25 healthcare workers, as of this writing, have become HIV positive as a result of occupational exposure. The risk of seroconversion, that is of becoming HIV positive, following a needlestick is less than 0.5%, compared with 12% risk of hepatitis B. There have been seroconversions following skin exposures to HIV-infected blood--and the same risk factors exist here as well, i.e. open wounds, skin ulceration, weeping dermatitis. For healthcare workers, the CDC has recommended uniform body substance precautions (complete protection against contact with any body substance) in essence meaning that all patients are considered infected with HIV. Avoidance of direct contact with potentially infected body substances is key. Extraordinary care is used to prevent injury by sharp instruments, both during their use and in their proper disposal. Even with the most stringent of protective protocols in place, four recent studies have established the rate of skin exposure to blood among operating room personnel at approximately 20%. In other words, nearly 1 in 5 of the personnel in an operating room will have direct contact with blood products.

Patients are afforded protection by high standards of sterilization policies and techniques utilized in medical facilities and by a sense of responsibility within the healthcare community supported by a number of national and state medical organizations for VOLUNTARY testing of healthcare workers.

What then are the "accepted" indications for antibody (HIV) testing?

      1.) For evaluation of blood and organs for tissue donation;

      2.) For those at risk by sexual transmission (sexual contact with homosexual men or unsafe heterosexual contacts) or a history of IV drug use;

      3.) For persons who received unscreened blood or factor concentrates after 1977;

      4.) For unexplained abnormalities in liver tests including positive hepatitis B markers;

      5.) For all persons with active tuberculosis;

      6.) And, for patients to whom healthcare workers have been exposed through injuries such as needlesticks.

The issue of the "right" of a patient to demand the results of his or her healthcare team's HIV testing or the "right" of a healthcare worker to refuse testing is not properly discussed in this forum. Most would acknowledge "rights" on "both sides of the fence." Most reasonable patients would acknowledge that if they are to make this demand of their physician or nurse, that they themselves must be willing to subject themselves to the same scrutiny and be tested. As "managed care" assumes a greater role in health care delivery, patients may be required to be tested for HIV on a regular basis. Most reasonable members of our society would acknowledge the need for ongoing research and budgeting proportionate to its benefits to society as a whole and unhurried by the political and emotional whirlwind surrounding this most devastating disease.

CHAPTER 28

PARTING SHOTS

Paradoxes of practicing medicine today.

The title of this chapter is a "play on words" of sorts, but there is accuracy in it as well. I plan on editorializing in this final chapter. Call it what you will, "artistic license", "author's option", but take it for what it is--an opportunity seized to educate you on the paradoxes in practicing medicine today. Like most shots, it may be painful initially. But a little pain for a greater good cannot be all bad.

My purpose is not to pose solutions, but only to stimulate thought. Society must continue to search for the best possible solutions. Through all of the statistics and rhetoric, we as physicians continue to come to work every day and face you, a "statistic". You should understand that we are continually barraged by the business and politics of medicine to abandon our primary bond to our patients. In this chapter, I fulfill my obligations to myself, to you as patients, and to my fellow physicians.

PARADOX 1: Self-Responsibility

One of the most obvious paradoxes as a physician I see every day is the patient who wants to be bailed out of a bad situation but has never done a thing to help him or herself to take simple, known measures to prevent the condition. I can't tell you how many legs are amputated from patients with vascular (blood vessel) problems, yet these patients have continued to smoke. In most cases this is the last of a long process, and almost invariably many times over they have been told to stop smoking--a habit which destines almost any treatment, including superb vascular procedures, to failure. Similarly, patients will subject themselves to back and joint surgeries carrying two or even three times their ideal body weight. Is it not unexpected that their own joints could not support the stresses of all this excess weight? Can they expect an artificial joint to perform any better?

In my practice, my bladder cancer patients continue to smoke despite being at very high risk for recurrence (more cancer) and being counseled on almost every office visit to "give 'em up". We continue to eat poorly despite being barraged in all forms of the media of its dangers--both short and long term. There is something almost subliminal at work here, and that is the basic failure of each of us to make ourselves accountable for our own well-being. It is as if health is something which should be "given" to us and compromising our health is something which "happens" to us, over which we have no control--as if we're passive in the whole process. With some diseases and accidents with injury, certainly this is the case. But venereal disease doesn't just happen, promiscuity allows it to happen. The choice to be promiscuous is an active choice. Far more common are health conditions which are the direct result of abusing this beautiful and amazingly intricate gift from the Almighty which we call the human body.

PARADOX 2: Accountability

A further paradox or twist to this notion of existing in a bubble and things happening to us is that while we are generally unwilling to be accountable to ourselves or to anyone else, we are very quick to be assured that there is accountability by someone else, especially through the legal system. This occurs most notably with a bad result. While certain diseases, conditions, or complications have well-studied and documented incidences, we are not accepting of them if we are the one who loses the leg or have a child with a birth defect. Physicians certainly should not be willing to accept that certain things "just happen", nor am I suggesting that outcomes or situations should not be scrutinized. I'm just saying that as a physician, I feel a need for society's legal, moral, ethical, and personal pendulum to swing back towards the middle. There needs to be a shared responsibility for health by the patient and the health care team. There needs to be more acceptance of less-than-perfect results by society but a sincere striving for excellence and improvement on the part of the medical community. There must be a recognition that health care, as we know it, is truly a misnomer. Current health care is reparative; it's damage control--mainly damage by the individual unto himself. True health care is preventative--instructive and nurturing of one's accountability to self in making day to day choices in living which affect the health of the individual and of society as a whole.

PARADOX 3: Cost Concerns

Pressures from government, employers, subscribers of health care, and even from within from hospitals and physicians dictate that medical care be run in a business-like manner. Programs are formulated to cover some conditions, not others, to cover some tests and procedures, not others, to utilize certain physicians and facilities, not others. In summary, these decisions are made to affect the bottom line--to move a potential loss situation to a gain or to improve the profit margin, like it or not. The strains on providing good "quality" care are real--the "quality" that we all expect because of our belief that human life is invaluable. We want to eliminate the skyrocketing costs in health care, yet if it's **my loved one** or **me** do whatever if necessary. There is ground to give on both sides, but what is absolutely necessary on both sides of the issue is the fidelity to the patient , the subscriber, the client (whatever term you wish to use for the human being) to whom we all pledge.

PARADOX 4: Technology-Driven

As a corollary to the above is that patients demand that the most up-to-date methods, techniques, and equipment be used for their care, yet they want to keep medical costs low. Someone has to pay for the $2.5 million lithotripter (stone crusher) in the basement of your hospital. Someone has to pay for the 5 to 10 years of intense laboratory and clinical research to put a new medication into use, estimated to be more than $350 million spent before even the first dose of a new medication is sold. The costs are spread across the board to all of us. Yet we abhor the cost of the hospital bed per day or the cost of an xray test using a $450,000 piece of equipment. The flip side of this issue is that every new technology does not need to replace time-tested techniques. Medicine is so very competitive that many times technology or science is touted simply as a means to give a certain hospital or physician(s) an edge over their competitors. Over time we find that the money spent has been wasted as the equipment settles into a use of very narrow indications. We all have paid the price for the hasty expenditure.

PARADOX 5: Government Involvement

The greatest of all paradoxes is the call for government to provide health care for all, yet a tremendous negativism and concern surfaces when one considers any business or venture which the government has entered in the past. As we shape our health care system of the future, one will not and cannot expect it to resemble or mimic the best of what we have today. Capitalism drives research and development, capitalism drives hospitals to be the best in their geographic area, and capitalism drives the health care team--physicians, nurses, therapists, and on and on. Extinguish capitalism from the health care system, and you will see many bright and good people exit the health care industry, hopefully to use their skills and expertise as contributors

241

in other areas, but certainly at our loss, as what could be more important than contributing to the health of individuals and to society at large?

The basis of socialism is the mindset that something is a "right" and government should provide that "right". Socialism breeds stagnation, a settling for mediocrity, and frustration for those who truly are pursuing excellence from which we can all benefit, whether at the laboratory bench or at the bedside. Capitalism need not poison one's conviction to the Hippocratic Oath which, in essence, promises fidelity to the good of another person as the prime aim. Capitalism without government interference need not be the enemy or prevent the accomplishing of the goals established by self-responsibility, accountability, and health care in its truest sense. Who gave government the assignment of providing this philosophical service, which really has more to do with basic attitudes than tangible goods? Have we forgotten that socialism has failed?

PARADOX 6: "Rights" and Responsibilities

With any "right" comes responsibility. If health care is a "right", then one has more than an accountability to him or herself to take better care of oneself through daily choices of a healthier lifestyle. If one chooses not to honor that responsibility, i.e. one chooses to smoke, or to be obese, or to ride motorcycles, or to speed in an automobile, or not see a physician annually if over age 50, or to have cocaine babies, then either that"right" is forfeited or a "pay as you play" mentality must be employed, i.e. cigarettes are $8.00 per pack with $6.00 going into the health care risk pool, or licensure for guns, motorcycles includes a fee for the risk pool, or the obese individual (there are specific medical criteria available) pay into the pool, or all alcoholic beverages are "taxed" according to alcohol content with those monies going to the risk pool, or moving violations in an automobile include a portion of the fine contributed to the risk pool. To not employ either of these two options, forfeiture or pay as you play, violates my rights as a responsible citizen honoring my responsibilities to myself and to a society supporting me.

PARADOX 7: Disclosure

Concerns regarding confidentiality infiltrate all levels of society today as computer technology allows the entry, storage, and retrieval of infinite bits of data on us all. Concerns regarding access to employment or health care as a result of retrievable medical records, criminal records, voting records, even

242

organizational membership records haunt us as much as being placed on"the list" in the McCarthy era. Society doesn't like this, and countless court proceedings exploring this area as a violation of confidentiality continue to redefine what is confidential and what is discoverable and usable. Yet as a physician, I am subject to a scrutiny well beyond that of John Doe, citizen. I must provide my medical history to my patients, even not-so-voluntarily subjecting myself to testing for a disease (AIDS) which they are less likely to contract in my operating room than by traveling in some of our major cities. Yet patients can refuse my request to discover that same disease in them. I am asked to relinquish my career if I test positive for AIDS, yet advocates admonish similar releases of AIDS patients in other workplaces. I must subject myself to data banks of my work performance, which on the surface are not supposed to be discoverable, yet in fact are; yet I must be extremely cautious in pursuing previous employers' work records when I function as a potential employer lest I violate the potential employee's confidentiality. Who has the right to and what is fair game for disclosure and discovery is continually being broadened.

PARADOX 8: Malpractice

If the loss of life and limb is priceless in the courts, so is it's preservation. That is what medicine does; it preserves life and limb. Yet we do, in fact, place values upon life and limb in the form of assigned values of reimbursement. The legal profession has escaped similar assignments, and in doing so has been a significant contributor to escalating health care costs. How so?

Settlements of suits or assignments of damages by juries have continued to rise, fueled by the simple fact that attorneys work on contingency and percentage, that is, they get paid if they win and on a percentage of what damages are won. This fuels the fire for more suits and pursuing of higher damages. There is little to discourage the use of the legal system as an avenue to pursue an instant, fully funded pension account!

What if the attorney had to collect a fee from his client and pay a fee to utilize the courts, whether the case was of merit or not, but involved our legal system, courts etc. This might discourage taking all comers and place some responsibility of payment upon the client as well as the attorney? What if we DRG'd (Diagnostic Related Groups, the equations used to determine physician reimbursement) the legal representation for loss of life or limb similar to what we do in for physician reimbursement? What if we pursued more vehemently quality review of use of our expensive courts by lawyers much like hospitals, insurance carriers, and even Uncle Sam do for physicians?

An important construct in the reshaping of health care in this country will by necessity be the addressing of the interfacing of the medical and legal disciplines. How we accomplish this and yet remain true to the inalienable rights of the individual will be our challenge.

SUMMARY

What weaves itself through all of the discussion of the paradoxes of practicing medicine and living good health in today's world is the fact that no matter how hard we try to employ basic tenets of other disciplines, whether it be scientific and technologic, business and financial, philosophical and theological, or political, medicine truly is unique. For while it takes from each in part, in total it transcends them all. It's what makes it so difficult to manage, yet it must be somehow to be workable in today's world; it's what makes it indispensable, yet so fragile and subject to destruction if significantly altered. It's what makes being a physician, in one and the same moment, the most wonderful and most frustrating profession.

GLOSSARY

Brief definition of key terms.

Author's Note: These definitions are tailored to the specific use(s) in this text. They are not intended or written to be all-encompassing. In other words, Webster should have no fear!

****

accommodation: process whereby the brain fails to read a constant incoming message. Also called habituation.
acquired immunodeficiency syndrome (AIDS): a disease of compromised or lost immune defenses.
anticholinergic: bladder relaxing effect.
autonomic nervous system: that portion of the nervous system which controls automatic functions, i.e. intestinal activity or bladder function.

behavior modification: treatment wherein certain activities or behaviors are altered to achieve a desired result, i.e. eliminating evening fluids for bedwetting.
benign: non-cancerous.
bladder: the hollow, muscular organ which serves to house and empty the urine.
bone scan: a nuclear medicine study in which a radioactive compound is administered and the bones are imaged; an important tool in metastatic evaluations.

calyx: a funnel-like structure delivering urine from the periphery into the central collection location of the kidney.
capacity: the volume capability, i.e. bladder capacity estimate in children (in ml) = (Age in years + 2) X 30; for adults, more variability, i.e. 250 to 450 ml.
caruncle: an abscess, or pus pocket, in the skin.

catheterization: placement of a drainage tube, i.e. a urethral or ureteral catheterization. In-and-out catheterization refers to placement, drainage, and removal in one setting.
chemotherapy: treatment for cancer in the form of medications.

cholinergic: bladder contracting effect.

chordee: the downward curvature of the penis, frequently associated with hypospadias.

circumcision: the surgical procedure the remove the excess foreskin of the penis.

clearance: the assessment of kidney filtration function.

colic: pain.

computerized axial tomography (CT Scan): special xray test using computer technology in which our internal organs and structures are viewed.

continence: control of bladder or bowel; also, dryness if the bladder has been removed, i.e. a continent urinary diversion.

corona: the circumferential groove just proximal to the head of the penis.

corpora cavernosa: the paired tubular chambers of the penis which become engorged to yield an erection. (Sing.: corpus cavernosum)

corpus spongiosum: the tubular structure on the underside of the penis which houses the urethra.

cryptorchidism: undescended testicle.

crystallization: the point beyond saturation which leads to formation of visible crystals by addition of the chemical in question, i.e. the crystallization of uric acid.

cyst: fluid-filled sack, usually benign in nature.

cystectomy: surgical removal of the bladder, i.e. radical cystectomy for cancer involves removal of the bladder and its attached structures with urinary diversion.

cystitis: infection of the bladder.

cystitis (interstitial): an inflammation of the bladder not of an infectious nature.

cystocoele: protrusion of the front wall of the vagina housing the back wall of the bladder.

cystometrogram (CMG): study of the bladder tone, performed through a catheter by the instillation of either water or carbon dioxide.

cystourethroscopy: a procedure wherein the bladder and urethra are viewed through special instruments either rigid or flexible.

detrusor: referring to the muscle of the bladder wall.

detumescence: the resolution of an erection.

dialysis: mechanical filtration process for assistance to failing kidney function.

dilation: a procedure to stretch or open, i.e. a urethral dilation with sounds.

diversion: the directing of urine away from the bladder by a surgical construction or placement of a drainage tube, i.e. an ileal loop following cystectomy.

diverticulum: pouch, or dog ear, i.e. bladder diverticulum.

double kidney: misnomer applied to a duplication of the ureters, with two ureters each of which drains a segment of the same kidney.

duplication: double, i.e. a ureteral duplication means two ureters draining the same kidney.

dysparunia: painful intercourse.

dyssynergia: bad synergy, two things are not working together as they should be but actually against each other, i.e. dyssynergia in Busy Little Girl Syndrome.

ejaculation: the jettisoning of sperm and secretions.

ejaculatory ducts: the location in the prostate from which the ejaculate is jettisoned.

electrocardiogram (EKG): heart tracing.

electromyogram (EMG): study of muscle activity, frequently performed upon the pelvic floor muscles in conjunction with a cystometrogram.

embryology: the study of formation of anatomic structures.

epididymis: the tubular structure attached to each testicle important for sperm maturation.

epididymorchitis: infection of the epididymis and testicle.

erectile dysfunction: the spectrum of disorders of penile erection, the end point of which is impotence.

extracorporeal shock wave lithotripsy (ESWL®): procedure of pulverization of kidney or ureteral stones by use of mechanical shock waves originating outside the body and directed by xray.

fascia: tough tissues over many muscles, particularly the abdominal wall which give strength and may be used for an incontinence procedure.

flow rate: the study determining the instantaneous rate of bladder emptying performed by voiding into a special flow urometer.

frenulum: the web of tissue on the underside of the penis in the midline which stretches from he shaft to the glans penis.

frequency: frequent urination.

furuncle: a collection of caruncles, or pus pockets, of the skin.

genitalia: external sex structures, i.e. penis and scrotum in males, labia and clitoris in females.

glans penis: the head of the penis.

glomerulus: the tuft or knot of blood vessels in the nephron where filtration of blood initially occurs.

habituation: the process whereby the brain phases out an incoming message which is constant and repeated. Also called accommodation.

hematuria: blood in the urine, either gross (visible) or microscopic (seen only under the microscope).

hernia: the protrusion of the belly cavity through a muscle weakness, typically thought of in the groin.

hesitancy: delay in initiating a urinary stream.

hormone: a chemical secreted by a gland which is distributed through the bloodstream and acts at a target organ for a specific function, i.e. LH results in testosterone production.

horseshoe kidney: a developmental formation of a kidney into the shape of a horseshoe.

human immunodeficiency virus (HIV): the causative virus for AIDS.

hydrocoele: fluid-filled sac in the scrotum.

hydronephrosis: dilated or stretched renal pelvis and associated collecting system structures.

hydroureteronephrosis: dilation or stretched ureter and collecting system of the kidney.

hypospadias: the congenital condition wherein the meatus or opening does not form at the tip of the penis.

hysterectomy: surgical removal of the female uterus.

idiopathic: of unknown cause, i.e. an idiopathic condition.

immunotherapy: treatment of cancer by enhancing the body's own immune (defense) system.

impotence: the inability to sustain an erection satisfactory for intercourse.

incontinence: lack of urinary or fecal control.

infection: contamination, usually by bacteria, which results in inflammation.

infertility: the state of being unable to procreate.

inflammation: swelling and pain resulting from and in irritation and/or infection.

intravenous pyelogram (IVP): an xray test involving injection of contrast to visualize the kidneys, ureters, and bladder.

introitus: the vaginal opening.

intromission: the introduction of the penis into the vagina during intercourse.

laparoscopy: the use of scopes to view the abdominal (peritoneal) cavity.

lithotripsy: pulverization of a stone, i.e. ESWL® or laser lithotripsy.

liver profile (function tests): blood tests to assess liver function; important in metastatic evaluations and assessments of overall health.

malignancy: cancer.

meatus: opening, usually referring to the opening of the urethra where urine exits.

medulla: central portion of the kidney.

metabolic: having to do with metabolism or our bodies' chemical reactions.

metastasis: spread outside of the site of origin, i.e. metastatic prostate cancer.

milliliter (ml.): a unit of volume measure, 5 ml equals one teaspoon. Also referred to as a cubic centimeter (cc.).

morbidity: harm, i.e. the morbidity of an illness.

mortality: death, i.e. the mortality of an illness.

multicystic kidney disease: disease of development in utero in which the kidneys form as a cluster of cysts with little to no function; thought to be a result of an early, complete or near-complete obstruction to kidney drainage.

nephron: the functional unit of the kidney.

nephroscopy: direct viewing of the kidney through special instruments.

nocturia: urinating during normal sleeping hours, usually nighttime.

nocturnal enuresis: bedwetting at night.

nocturnal penile tumescence (NPT): the study of the ability of the penis to achieve erection during sleep.

oligohydramnios: a smaller amount than normal of fluid bathing the fetus.

orgasm: the perceived achieving of sexual climax.

orifice: an opening or hole, i.e. the ureteral orifice in the bladder where urine is extruded from the kidney.

papilla: a mound-like structure in the kidney containing the final lengths of nephrons.

parenchyma: the functional or "meat" portion of the kidney.

paraphimosis: foreskin retraction behind the head of the penis with constriction and inability to be retracted back over the penile head.

parasympathetic nervous system: autonomic nervous system involved with erection and bladder emptying.

pelvic kidney: a kidney residing in the true pelvis, rather than in its normal location.

pelvis: the funnel-like collecting structure of the kidney which directs the urine into the ureter. Also, the lower abdomen area housing the bladder, rectum, and female structures.

penis: the tubular male organ for sexual functon and urination.

percutaneous: through the skin, i.e. percutaneous nephroscopy.

peritoneal cavity: the sac or cavity in which our intestines reside.

peristalsis: the smooth, coordinated contraction of a smooth muscled organ, i.e. the ureter or intestine.

Peyronie's Disease: an idiopathic condition of penile curvature and lump(s).

phimosis: the condition of adherence of redundant foreskin over the head (glans) of the penis preventing good hygiene and viewing for self-examination.

polycystic kidney disease: inherited disorder of kidney failure resulting from complete engulfment of the kidney with cysts; infantile type is autosomal recessive inheritance, adult type is autosomal dominant inheritance.

posterior urethral valves: leaflets of tissue in the prostate of some infants which obstruct with urination due to billowing like the wind in a sail.

procreate: to bear offspring.

prostate gland: the accessory sex gland involved in the production of sexual secretions and in bladder protection from infection.

prostate hyperplasia: benign (non-cancerous) enlargement of the prostate gland.

prostate hypertrophy: also benign (non-cancerous) enlargement of the prostate gland.

prostatectomy: removal of the prostate; radical prostatectomy includes removal of the prostate, seminal vesicles, and portions of the vas deferens.

prostatic specific antigen (PSA): a special blood test for the early detection of prostate cancer.

prostatitis: infection of the prostate gland.

prostatodynia: pain from the prostate, usually in chronic prostatitis.

prosthesis: man-made device, i.e. penile prosthesis for erections or artificial sphincter prosthesis for anti-incontinence.

pyelogram: xray of the kidney.

pyelonephritis: infection of the kidney

pyuria: pus cells, or white blood cells, in the urine.

radiation therapy: the treatment of cancer by directed xray beam.

rectocoele: a protrusion of the back wall of the vagina housing the rectum.

referred pain: pain felt at a different location than the insult usually due to shared nerves by development, i.e. referred pain to the penis from prostate irritation.

reflux (vesicoureteral): pathologic condition in which urine tracks back up the ureter, occasionally up to the kidneys, during urination serving as a source of infection.

renal: referring to the kidney.

renal cell carcinoma: cancer of the parenchyma (meat portion) of the kidney.

renal pelvis: the funnel-like structure conducting urine from the kidney into the ureter.

residual: the volume of urine remaining in the bladder upon completion of urination.

retrograde pyelogram: xray of the kidney performed by injection contrast backward from the bladder to the kidney through the ureteral orifice.

saturation: the point at which no further absorption or concentration can be performed without crystal formation, i.e. the saturation of a chemical in urine.

scrotum: the sac-like structure of the male genitalia which houses the testicles.

sebaceous cyst: small ball-like structure in the skin consisting of a collection of fluid normally secreted by the sweat glands associated with a hair follicle.

semen: the secretions jettisoned during ejaculation which includes sperm and the secretions of the prostate gland and seminal vesicles.

seminal vesicles: two accessory sex glands which attach to the prostate gland and are responsible for approximately 50% of the ejaculate.

smooth muscle: a special type of muscle which works by slow deliberate contraction, like a worm's motion, rather than sudden jerk-like motion, i.e. the muscle of the bladder or of the intestine.

sounds: instruments passed through the urethra for dilation of a stenosis.

sperm: the individual cell for procreation; sometimes used as individual or cumulatively, the latter is more accurately called semen if it includes the other sex secretions.

spermatocoele: sperm-filled cyst on the epididymis.

sphincter: a muscle for closure of an aperture, i.e. the urinary sphincters for continence; also, the artificial prosthesis which provides the same function.

stenosis: tightening or narrowing leading to blockage, i.e. urethral stenosis.

sterile: free from infection or contamination; also, unable to procreate.

stress incontinence: leakage of urine with lifting and straining.

stricture: a narrowed or constricted area generally causing problems by obstruction to flow, i.e. a urethral stricture.

sympathetic nervous system: an autonomic nervous system involved in blood pressure control, ejaculation, and bladder sphincter control.

synergy: two things added together yielding a greater result than their simple additive effect, i.e. the synergy of voiding.

testicle (testes): the male organ of sperm and testosterone production located in the scrotum.

torsion: twisting, i.e. torsion of the testicle.

transplantation: the placement of an organ, i.e. kidney, into position for function.

transitional cell cancer: cancer of this "skin" type which may occur at any of its sites including the kidney, ureter, bladder, prostate, and part of the urethra.

transitional cell epithelium: the "skin" lining of the bladder, ureter, and renal pelvis.

trigone: triangular area at the bladder neck, the three points of which are the two ureteral orifices and the bladder outlet; significant for its concentration of sensory nerves.

TULIP: transurethral laser incision of prostate.

TUMP: transurethral microwave prostatectomy.

tumor markers: blood tests used as indicators of the presence of caner, i.e. PSA for prostate, AFP and B-HCG for testes cancer.

TURBT: transurethral resection of bladder tumor.

TURP: transurethral resection of prostate.

tumescence: erection.

ultrasound: study of architecture by bouncing painless sound ways off of a structure and the echo yields an image.

United Network For Organ Sharing (UNOS): the national system for organ donation and candidacy for transplantation.

ureter: the muscular tube which conducts the urine from the kidney to the bladder.

ureterocoele: a sac-like dilation of the ureter in the bladder resulting from a partial blockage at its meatus.

ureteropelvic junction: the joining of the renal pelvis with the ureter and a site for constriction.

UPJ obstruction: blockage, partial or complete, at the juncture of the ureter with the renal pelvis.

ureteroscopy: a direct look into the ureter through special flexible or rigid scopes.

ureterovesicle junction: the joining of the ureter with the bladder and a site for constriction or reflux.

urethra: the hollow tube conducting the urine from the bladder to the outside.

urethritis: infection of the urethra, i.e. nonspecific urethritis.

urge incontinence: urinary leakage associated with urgency.

252

urgency: sudden, strong sensation to urinate.

urinalysis: the chemical and microscopic analysis of a urine specimen.

urination: the act of emptying the bladder's contents.

urine: the liquid produced by the kidneys containing wastes and excess fluids from our blood.

urine culture: a special test in which bacteria contained within infected urine are grown in the laboratory for identification and testing of antibiotic sensitivity.

urodynamics: term to encompass the testing of the tone and emptying ability of the bladder, i.e. CMG, EMG, flow rate, and residual.

urolithiasis: urinary stones

Urologist: a surgical specialist dealing in disorders of the adrenal glands, kidneys, ureters, bladder, prostate, seminal vesicles, and male genitalia.

vaginitis: infection of the female vagina.

varicocoele: dilated veins in the scrotum, typically on the left side.

vas deferens: the muscular tube conducting sperm from the epididymis to the ejaculatory duct in the prostate.

vasectomy: the procedure of male sterilization in which the vas deferens are occluded.

vasopressin: water conserving, blood vessel constricting.

venereal: sexually transmitted.

voiding cystourethrogram (VCUG): study of the bladder emptying by filling it with contrast and observing voiding with xray.

Wilm's Tumor: a special type of kidney cancer almost exclusively in children.

254

INDEX

transitional cell epithelium, 110
transplantation, *161*
transurethral laser incision of the
    prostate (TULIP), 51
transurethral microwave
    prostatectomy (TUMP), 51
transurethral resection of a bladder
    tumor (TURBT), 112
transurethral resection of the prostate
    (TURP), 52
trichomoniasis, *233*
trigone, 41, 75, *144*
tubal ligation, 196
tuberculosis (TB), 109

—U—

ultrasound
    prostate gland, 57
    testicular, 190
undescended testicle, 189
United Network for Organ Sharing
    (UNOS), *163*
ureter, 75, 119, *142*
ureteropelvic junction obstruction,
    122
ureteroscopy, *133*
urethra, 26, 75
    prostatic, 40, 44
urethral stenosis, 91
urethritis
    nonspecific, *229*
urinary incontinence, 71
    stress, 79
urinary retention, 47

urinary sphincter, 72
uroflow, 48
urologist, 3

—V—

varicocoele, *175*, 188
    infertility, 206
vas deferens, 42
vasectomy, 195
    infertility, 208
    procedure, 199
vasovasostomy, 208
venereal disease, 227
    genital ulcer, *228*
    gonorrhea, *227*
    Hepatitis B, *232*
    herpes, *231*
    lice and mites, *233*
    molluscum contagiosum (MCV),
        232
    nonspecific urethritis, *229*
    trichomoniasis, *233*
    warts, *230*
Venous Leak Syndrome, 9
vesicoureteral reflux, 127, 214

—W—

Wilm's Tumor, *131*

—Z—

Zoladex®, 68